REGENERATING SEXUAL POTENTIAL

Revolutionary Treatment
Solutions for Sexual
Dysfunction Using
Platelet-Rich Plasma (PRP)

BY LISBETH ROY, D.O.

Regenerating Sexual Potential: Revolutionary Treatment Solutions for Sexual Dysfunction Using Platelet-Rich Plasma (PRP)

Printed in the United States
BOOK PRODUCTION DESIGN: T.L. Price • design@tlpricefreelance.com

Dedication

This book is dedicated to my patients. Thank you all so much for your confidence and your appreciation of my art. Without your willingness to teach and to allow the exploration of ideas, there would be no book. In fact, without your willingness to participate, there would be no advancement at all.

A special thanks to all who contributed your voices, stories and experience both to this book and through your participation in the many physician training sessions.

You are the reason I continue to seek opportunities to learn and to apply what I have learned. You are the passion that is so obvious to all when I speak about our experience with the technology of platelet rich plasma.

Lisbeth Roy

TABLE OF CONTENTS

Part 4. Physiological Causes of Sexual Dysfunction **171**

Chapters 11: Hormonal Changes as a Cause of Sexual Dysfunction 173

Chapters 12: Sexual Changes Should be Considered "The Canary in the Cave." They are Often the First Symptom of a Serious Disease. 185

Chapters 13: Many Medications Can Cause Noticeable Changes in Sexual Function............................ 193

Chapters 16: Why Do Men Grow Breasts and Women Grow Mustaches? How Men and Women are Hormonally Similar and What Happens When the Balance is Tipped in the Wrong Direction

Chapters 17: How Nutrition and Supplements Make a Difference in Enhancing Sexual Function and Experience

Chapters 18: Is the "Little Blue Pill" All There Is?

Chapters 22: PRP & Other Options for Incontinence Treatment 273

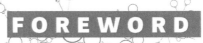

FOREWORD

As a board certified Urologist who has specialized in sexual medicine for over 35 years, I truly believe that this book should resonate with and stimulate both patients and clinicians alike.

I serve as an assistant professor of surgery at the University of Illinois, and I am active in the education of medical students and family practice residents. Over the years, I've treated thousands of patients for sexual dysfunction and incontinence. Unfortunately, only a few patients are actually *cured* of their primary disease. This is because most practitioners practice tertiary medicine. However, the educational process now leans towards intercepting the disease, which is in stark contrast to the way medicine was taught just a few years ago.

Today, modern medicine focuses more on prevention, decreasing the terrible sequelae that can occur. This is the corner stone of Dr. Roy's practice and PRP therapy.

Three years ago, I met Dr. Lisbeth Roy at the Annual Sexual Medicine Society. It was obvious to me she had a real passion for her patients using Platelet Rich Plasma (PRP). I was intrigued to learn more about PRP therapy and, before the end of the meeting, we scheduled training at my facility. Being a Urologist in sexual medicine, PRP seemed to be a promising adjunct to the various treatment modalities already in place.

At that time, Dr. Roy and I discussed the animal studies supporting PRP in sexual dysfunction, and decided clinical studies in human patients were desperately needed.

As a Functional Medicine Physician, Dr. Roy's goal is to achieve a total solution for her patients. Her devotion to sexual wellness and regenerative therapy is clearly defined in this text. The dynamics surrounding sexual dysfunction affect more than half of the worlds' population, and undoubtedly you know someone who is devastated by this affliction.

Within this book, Dr. Roy helps you to understand PRP and the importance of hormonal balance and optimal cellular function. The nutritional changes coupled with behavioral modification is monumental in alleviating diseases such as diabetes, hypertension and lipid disorders. She has compiled basic science along with observations to fully explain the disease process and the risk of not seeking treatment.

Dr. Roy's magnetic voice can draw anyone near to listen, and her attentiveness to respond is respectful and gentle. She is brilliant and empathetic; is a true pioneer and trailblazer for the PRP movement!

I've found that her certified PRP procedure trainings provide a real knowledge for physicians and clinicians. After attending her workshop, clinicians walk away with a better understanding of the disease process and how PRP can facilitate the patients' treatment plan.

Dr. Roy is my mentor and close friend. Her perseverance and commitment to the advancement of PRP has changed the way I practice medicine in 2016. PRP clinical trials are coming later in the year to prove the observations we've seen to date.

Joseph J. Banno   Assistant Clinical Professor, University of Illinois Peoria School of Medicine · Senior Partner Midwest Urological Group

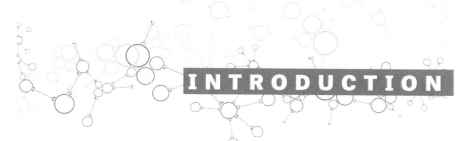

Thank you for choosing to read this book. I can assure you that there are new concepts introduced that really change the playing field when it comes to successfully treating sexual dysfunction, urinary incontinence and beyond.

Let me talk about "**improved tissue potential**" right away so that you will have a foundation upon which to apply all of the additional suggested treatment options. I know this sounds a bit scientific, but it's a simple approach that changes the context of all treatment discussions. We are moving into an age when "Regenerative Medicine" is not just a notion, but an affordable reality. The landscape is changing rapidly and the advancements will likely reach each one of us during our lifetime.

Platelet Rich Plasma (PRP) improves tissue potential. The tissues of the body contain receptors upon which hormones and nutrients cause an effect. As tissues age they lose the responsiveness or "potential" to respond.

When you successfully regenerate and rejuvenate this tissue, you are improving its potential to react to chemical stimuli (hormones, neurotransmitters, nutrients and even medication chemicals). It only makes sense that if a patient is to have the most effective treatment strategy, regenerating potential is first line therapy. Why would you go through the trouble of optimizing hormones, changing diet, and addressing other imbalances if you do not also improve the body's ability to respond to such intervention?

The next concept is that both sexual dysfunction and urinary incontinence are "**progressive diseases**". This simply means that they get worse if not treated effectively. Treatment should be sought sooner rather than later if total resolution is to be achieved. Total resolution or "rehabilitation" is relatively new in the sexual dysfunction and urinary incontinence discussion. Total rehabilitation is very possible and should be the goal of treatment.

I am trained in natural bio-identical hormone therapy and have completed extensive training in anti-aging, functional, sexual and regenerative medicine as a fellow in Anti-Aging, Functional & Regenerative Medicine and a fellow in Stem Cell Therapies through The American Academy of Anti-Aging Medicine (A4M).

The goal for my practice is to help patients achieve optimal health and wellness at all ages, to slow or reverse the symptoms and diseases often associated with aging, to enhance the quality of life and increase cellular potential. The problems discussed in this book affect fifty percent of the male and female population. We are growing older in a lesser state of peak performance and need to help educate people of the possibility of aging well -and functioning optimally.

We have a great deal of control over our state of wellness. Disease does not just happen; it takes years of cellular changes and symptom development before the threshold of disease is reached. Many people do not feel well, but because they are not yet diseased, most physicians have no treatment to offer.

I provide patients with complete evaluation and exploration to the causes of their symptoms. Once the imbalances are identified and corrected, wellness is re-established and disease is diverted. Disease is opportunistic and cannot exist in a well-balanced body.

As a regenerative medicine practitioner, I feel that regenerative approaches offer the highest yield with regard to the potential of a successful wellness strategy. Really, you can feed and aid a degenerating system, or you can implement treatments that actually turn back the clock and provide ideal function.

I have many patients who seek my expertise because they feel well but may have challenging family medical histories and do not wish to be the next one affected by the 'inherent diseases'. Most people do not realize that their family history is important, because it identifies their physiologic "weak link." Identifying this weak link gives opportunity to strengthen it, thus raising the level of wellness and again diverting the opportunity for disease. For example, if your family has a strong predisposition for adult onset diabetes, you can be spared the challenge of the disease by eating only whole fresh foods, drinking clean water, getting moderate exercise and balancing your hormones. This provides your body the nutrients necessary for insulin cell signaling and keeps the cells receptive.

Ninety-seven percent of all the money spent on healthcare (more than $70 billion each year) is paid to support people who have diseases that are preventable, such as adult onset diabetes, cardiovascular disease and even cancer. I personalize a strategy for each patient to keep his or her body healthy and maintain a youthful zest for life with every aging year.

Most of us are not afraid of aging, we just don't want to *feel* old. I have many patients in their later years that look and feel great. Age is not the problem, the state of wellness is what dictates the quality of life. There are many 30 to 50-year-old people who are relatively young, but they feel fatigued, unmotivated, unhappy, and generally unwell without recognizing the true cause.

For a great deal of people, "getting old" is defined as changes in appearance, energy, well-being, sexual interest and sexual function. We often joke that hearing is the second thing to go as we age... implying that sexual function is the first. A man may not be bothered by his graying hair, but his ability to perform sexually is part of his core definition of what it means to be "a man." A woman might accept some laugh lines with grace, but a lack of desire and intimacy can leave her feeling unattractive, old, or "used up". Sexual changes often interfere with partner intimacy. The decline in function or desire can be misinterpreted and thus mistaken for a lack of interest or worse, a lack of attractiveness.

Preserving sexual function, or even reversing the sexual aging process, is often about balancing hormones and the health of the sexual system. I am not just looking at how we can "mix things up in the bedroom." Many couples are madly in love and are adventurous, but their physiology (or physical response) is what's failing. I propose that we have safe and effective treatments available right now that enhance overall sexual potential from a **biological perspective**. This is a leading-edge concept, and it is my hope to champion its cause in my practice -and now on a greater scale, through this book.

First, please know that in spite of everything you may have been told, **it is possible to improve your health and sexual well-being**. You may have just recently noticed a change in your sexual desire, performance, pleasure or your ability to please your partner. You may be suffering in silence and debilitated by the challenges you face in achieving satisfying sexual function. No matter what stage or frustration you are in, there is help and even the possibility of full recovery.

The treatment strategies can range from prevention and preservation of sexual capabilities to full rehabilitation. Of course my first choice as a Functional Medicine Physician is to preserve and treat early for the best results.

Approximately 50 percent of all men and women report some degree of sexual dysfunction that interferes with their quality of life. This is a staggering problem for a large segment of the population, and it demands a strong solution – a biological solution. In my practice, we offer a comprehensive approach that goes well beyond the one-size-fits-all strategy of prescription medication alone.

Prescribing pills for men or lubrication for women and allowing them to believe that the loss of sexual desire and/or function is "simply a part of the aging process" doesn't necessarily solve their problem. Instead, I strive to help my patients understand and overcome the signs and symptoms of "getting old" by helping them restore balance and true physiological changes.

It is my experience that with education and medical innovations, we can maintain health and youthfulness into our golden years and beyond. I work with my patients to develop nutritional plans and healthy living strategies that, combined with medical treatments, will help them be active, vital, and youthful at any age.

Know this: there are solutions to sexual dysfunction for men and women, and this book contains a detailed approach for both. I understand how changes in sexual response can affect relationships. Men can identify the source of their problems more easily than women, because there is no way to hide their sexual challenges. Everyone in the bedroom knows when a man is unable to achieve and maintain an erection and there is no way of hiding premature ejaculation (PE). Conversely, depending on the severity of a woman's dysfunction, she can still engage in sexual relations even if she no longer desires to or even if she does not gain any pleasure from it. She may never identify that there is a problem as long as she can continue to meet the needs of her partner.

There are many good physical and psychological reasons to rejuvenate and preserve sexual activity. The intimacy during the sexual experience is absolutely essential for a healthy relationship. It is the very thing that makes the relationship with your partner different from others. Think about it...there's a spring in your step after a night of sharing intimacy, correct? Sexual intimacy is relationship glue! Sexual satisfaction and comfort are pleasures of being human.

Ignoring sexual dysfunction will also have a negative impact on self-esteem. While men are often motivated to repair sexual problems, women unfortunately come up short in this area. In fact, women might often sense there is a strain or change in the relationship without correctly identifying that the change in intimacy could be the cause -rather than a symptom. This is largely because sexual dysfunction happens more subtly for women. Sometimes women blame themselves for a lack of desire or sexual response. They don't realize chemical and other physiologic changes occur that are beyond their control. Correcting these imbalances and employing a regenerative strategy is the right answer to restoring the whole human experience.

To compound the problem, when a woman does discuss sexual problems with her doctor she is often given inadequate information and therefore, offered little help. Most physicians are not knowledgeable or even skilled in this area and often do not view sexual changes as "real" problems. Many physicians never think about the physiological reasons why these symptoms are present. All symptoms tell the story of physiologic changes that may even be the precursor to "real" disease.

As hormone levels change, there's also a change in desire. Add to that the stressors of everyday life and you have a recipe for simply not being interested. I see this every day. A new patient may admit to a decline in libido, but unless there is pressure at home, she will often not be concerned about a solution. She does not realize the impact on her psyche and possibly the impact on her relationship that's at risk. Women have to advocate for themselves and thus be proactive — even relentless — in seeking help.

WHY do women commonly allow their sexual self to just fade away? It is betrayal to themselves and to their partners. As a woman and a physician, I feel it is a mistake to allow this to happen. Sexual intimacy is one of the ways we find balance in our lives. It is one of the ways we get to know ourselves and bond with our partner. No matter what you think or have been taught to think about sex — sexuality and sexual intimacy is important.

After starting treatment with a female patient, inevitably, she returns a few weeks later grateful for helping her to remember how important it is to feel attractive and sexually alive. She reports that her relationship is better along with her health in general. How easy it is to forget the impact sexual health has on the quality of life.

The symptoms of sexual dysfunction and urinary incontinence deserve to be treated with attention and concern.

In the recent past, treatment options have been limited. This is no longer the case. We have non-surgical options that can effectively restore libido, vaginal lubrication, sensitivity, intensity of orgasm and resolve urinary incontinence. We can help men achieve firmer erections, improved sensitivity, have more intense orgasms and enhanced sexual stamina. **If any of that sounds desirable, this book was written for you.**

My goal is be an advocate for a comprehensive review of various strategies that can be used to improve sexual function– strategies that I have had significant success with in my practice. The most exciting solution comes from advancements made in using Platelet Rich Plasma (PRP) to treat sexual dysfunction and urinary incontinence. This medical procedure has advanced other medical practices by leaps and bounds and is now the most innovative tool on the market.

PRP is an autologous procedure and involves drawing blood, concentrating the platelets and strategically injecting them back into the body to regenerate tissues. The procedures are simple, safe and effective. They change the playing field, because they actually regenerate and rejuvenate sexual organs and erogenous zones at a cellular level. The regeneration and rejuvenation process leads to improved sexual potential for all individuals. By incorporating PRP treatments with traditional therapies, I've been able to customize solutions for patients and restore sexual function in some of the most severe cases.

Note that changes in sexual function can be a harbinger for anything from hormone imbalances to cardiovascular problems. Consulting your general doctor is an important first step, but it might become necessary to speak with an expert in the field. Take the initiative, seek proper care in anti-aging, functional, and regenerative medicine. Ensure that he or she has special training in restoring sexual function using PRP and knows how to layer other technologies for synergistic effect and benefit. A specially trained physician can help you achieve your goals and find the right solution for you.

It is my passion and hope that PRP procedures will soon be included in all solution protocols and will become a new standard of care in treating male and female sexual dysfunction and incontinence. However, a focus needs to be placed on PRP procedures for doctors to master and for patients to request the treatment.

My vision for this book:

- Improve the delivery of care to patients with sexual dysfunction and urinary incontinence.

- Raise awareness to the progressive nature and severity of sexual function and incontinence in terms of short-term and long-term consequence. Champion the truth that rehabilitation is possible using PRP/BHRT/ICP and other options.

- Encourage the practice of rehabilitation and prevention by keeping the sexual process active.

- Encourage doctors and patients that urgent intervention of these progressive processes offer better outcomes than traditional treatments. Raise awareness that comprehensive treatment approaches are highly effective at rehabilitating, regenerating and rejuvenating the sexual system.

- Advance the technology of PRP and its benefits for sexual wellness and incontinence.

- Educate patients to pursue a complete evaluation and comprehensive treatment strategy to ensure restoration of optimal function and wellness.

Providing these procedures to patients has been an amazing opportunity for me as a doctor. While I want to expand this offering to more patients, I also want to enlighten physicians across the country about this safe and effective medical solution. As a result, this book is written for patients and physicians alike, but I will seek to explain and simplify medical terminology so it is easily digestible by all readers.

I am pleased that you are accompanying me on this journey as we explore the challenges of sexual dysfunction, non-invasive solutions and break-through treatments that offer the possibility of full rehabilitation.

This book is broken down into five sections so you can easily navigate the chapters that will be of most value to you. Let it empower you to take action; to fully participate in your own sexual wellness. Let it serve as a guide so that you can become an advocate for your own sexual health and enjoy intimacy again.

- **Part One:** A "Real" Regenerative Breakthrough in Sexual Medicine of the 21st Century: O-Shot™ and Priapus Shot™
- **Part Two:** The Importance of Being a Sexual Being...and you thought it was just for fun!
- **Part Three:** Defining and Refining Sexual Function and Sexual Pleasure
- **Part Four:** Physiologic Causes of Sexual Dysfunction
- **Part Five:** How Other Treatments can Layer with PRP Technology to Improve Sexual Function and Pleasure
- **Part Six:** How Incontinence Impacts Quality of Life and Independent Living & How PRP Can Help

Above all, please never lose interest or hope. Many of my patients have been forever changed by the progressive approach to wellness that I have defined in this book.

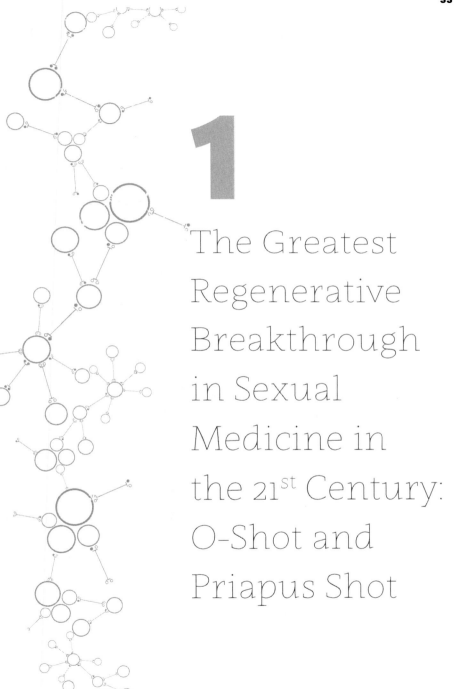

1

The Greatest Regenerative Breakthrough in Sexual Medicine in the 21st Century: O-Shot and Priapus Shot

Platelet Rich Plasma (PRP) therapy has been around for decades, but the attention it is receiving has only recently begun to reach appropriate heights. PRP therapy is revolutionizing multiple areas of medicine, from wound care and repair of nerve/muscle damage to cosmetic medicine and even hair growth. But to me, PRP is simply the most exciting breakthrough in sexual medicine — ever.

The O-Shot™ for women and Priapus Shot™ for men are non-surgical, simple, pain-free treatments that restore sexual vitality and improve sexual well-being by leveraging the body's natural ability to heal itself. If that sounds too good to be true, read on — I promise this technology has the potential to change your life.

CHAPTER 1

The Technology of Platelet Rich Plasma

You know your body can regenerate itself. You continuously grow new skin and hair, you produce new blood cells, and even your bones will mend on their own when set in place and protected by a cast. PRP therapy works by focusing that natural healing ability on specific regions of your body that you would like to heal or rejuvenate.

Doctors achieve this by removing whole blood from the patient and processing it through specialized kits to remove just the platelet rich plasma (PRP). The patient's PRP, created from his or her own blood, is injected strategically to accelerate the body's natural healing and regenerative process. The regenerative process slows down as we age. Cells die and functions diminish. Injecting activated PRP is like turning the process back on; it's turning back the clock and turning on rejuvenation.

There are two methods of PRP preparation approved by the US Food & Drug Administration (FDA); both processes involve taking whole blood and sending it through two stages of centrifugation designed to separate the PRP aliquot from platelet-poor plasma and red blood cells. Platelet Rich Plasma treatments have been used as a clinical tool for decades across several types of medical treatments. However, you have probably never heard of PRP until recent years and only then if you're a huge sports fan. Over the last several years, PRP therapy has received a great deal of attention in the press for its use in treating sports injuries, particularly those of high-profile professional athletes (Schwarz 2009).

PRP treatments have been used for years to improve the healing process of wounds and the success of bone grafting surgeries. Within the last ten years, PRP has been used for treating common orthopedic-related sports conditions involving muscle and tissue damage with great success. In 2009, research showed promise in using platelet-rich plasma as catalysis for bone repair to improve healing and shorten recovery time (**www.news-medical.net**). Since then, major sports figures have been very public about using PRP treatments.

In 2011, NBA guard Brandon Roy announced his retirement from the Portland Trailblazers. His reasons were based on persistent issues with both of his knees. After six knee surgeries, he no longer had any cartilage remaining in his joints and doctors advised him to stop playing. But in 2012, he announced his comeback. What happened to cause the dramatic turnaround? *PRP therapy* (Niesen 2012)!

Kobe Bryant of the LA Lakers also reportedly sought PRP treatment in Germany in 2011 to help him deal with lingering problems with an arthritic joint in his right knee (Niesen 2012). It has also been used by other sports stars such as Dwight Howard, Tiger Woods, Ray Lewis and Peyton Manning for a wide-variety of reasons (Carroll 2013).

In baseball, pitchers Dylan Bundy and Jonny Venters used PRP injections for rehab after surgery. Athletes such as Alex Rodriguez, Chris Britton and Zach Greinke received incredible results with PRP injections without surgery (Carroll 2013). And while anecdotal evidence is abundant in sports medicine, there have been significant scientific findings as well. One of the most impressive was published in the American Journal of Sports Medicine's 2013 edition detailing a study led by Dr. Luga Podesta.

Dr. Podesta found that eighty-eight percent of athletes in his study returned to "work" (play) without further need of surgery after receiving PRP treatments. The study also documented physical changes inside the elbow (his focus of research) thereby disproving the placebo effect. Another study published in the same journal this year documented proof that PRP was more effective than placebo injections for knee osteoarthritis (Patel 2013).

In a 2009 article, Dr. Lindsay Harris and Andrew I. Larson of the Aspen Orthopedic Associates and Aspen Sports Medicine Foundation explained how PRP treatment can accelerate healing of damaged tissue (Harris 2009). In the treatment of musculoskeletal diseases and injuries, PRP has been used to initiate the body's healing response within damaged tissue. This offered doctors an alternative when treating sports injuries.

As early as 2008, the Pittsburg Steelers' wide receiver, Hines Ward, received PRP for a knee medial collateral ligament sprain and was a pivotal member of his team as they went on to win the Super Bowl. Ward credited PRP treatment for his ability to play in that game and his resulting success was covered in the national media.

So, as you can see, PRP treatments are making headlines all over the world in sports medicine!

But PRP benefits extend far beyond this area of medicine with amazing results in a wide-range of therapeutic areas. In fact, I worked with a cosmetic dentist who said she could not do her job if it were not for PRP. Her patients have deteriorating bones with slow healing tissues. She is charged with implanting, repairing and regenerating her patients' dental features for improved wellness, and she claims without PRP, the work would rarely be success-ful. PRP technology helps regrow bone, ligament and soft tissue. Repairs are successful and long lasting.

PRP therapy is being used in at least a dozen therapeutic areas and it's very exciting to advance its use in achieving sexual wellness and urinary continence. For individuals who have experienced various forms of muscle, nerve, or tissue damage, PRP treatments can correct sexual dysfunction. It can also help men and women with mediocre sexual function to respond better to stimulation because treatments improve sensitivity and arousal. In short, PRP therapy is heaven sent — or at least mother-nature sent — for individuals who want to maintain healthy sex lives at any age!

This book is not just an advertisement for PRP therapy. I want you to really understand how PRP works and why it is a safe and effective tool. Therefore, in the sections ahead, I will review the fundamentals of PRP, how it works, and the science behind the medicine.

What is PRP Treatment?

Platelet-Rich Plasma (PRP) therapy is a method that uses the patient's own blood and, through a processing system, yields high levels of platelets. These platelets contain growth factors to accelerate the body's natural healing and regenerative process. When doctors use PRP procedures in medical treatments, they are increasing the concentration of platelets in the blood above their baseline levels, thus increasing the platelet's associated growth factors. The literature clearly shows regenerative benefits to tissues that receive treatment with 4-6 times baseline platelet concentration, or more specifically, 1.0 - 1.5 million platelet concentration.

The clinical benefit of PRP has been explored in several medical treatments, including the following:

- Healing of musculoskeletal tissues
- Repair of nerve damage/injuries
- Repair of muscle damage/injuries
- Bone repair
- Plastic/cosmetic surgery
- Oral surgery

- Wound care
- Hair regrowth
- Facial rejuvenation
- Dry eye resolution

Scientific data supports PRP proving it's beneficial in enhancing cell migration and cell proliferation, thus facilitating regeneration of tissue. Advancements have also been made in treating and repairing various connective tissue structures as well as regrowth of new nervous and vascular tissues. This regenerative action is what proves beneficial in improving penile function, increasing genital sensitivity, ease of orgasm, arousal and often resolving incontinence.

PRP stimulates stem cells located in the treatment area to grow new tissue. PRP is also the fertilizer for the regenerative process thus supplying many growth and healing factors. Newly regenerated tissue has increased potential. This means that it has the opportunity to work better because it is a newer tissue; it can receive hormones, nutrients and even medications with improved action. New tissue has greater potential than degenerated tissue.

The Treatment Process

During the PRP Treatment Process, blood is drawn from the patient and placed in a special processing unit that separates platelets, white blood cells and serum from red blood cells. The white blood cells and platelets are concentrated and collected into a sterile syringe. Calcium Chloride is then added to the PRP to signal activation, thereby releasing growth factors and healing elements into the area being treated.

When these small amounts of highly concentrated platelets are injected into the damaged area of the body, the delivery of growth factors and healing enzymes facilitate the body's ability to grow new soft tissue and/or bone cells. Because PRP can be activated, or tricked into thinking there is an injury in a non-injured area, it can deliver the healing instincts of platelets, leading to regeneration of tissue and therefore an improvement in function.

Before PRP is injected, local anesthetic is administered to the skin and soft tissue where the patient receives the treatment. Depending on the size of the injured tissue/area, multiple injections can be used in order to optimize the treatment effectiveness.

PRP injections are administered with small gaged needles. When combined with numbing agents, patients report the treatment is pain-free — even when being administered in highly sensitive areas such as the vagina or penis.

Research and clinical data demonstrates that PRP injections are extremely safe for the patient, with minimal risk of complication. Also, because PRP is created from the patient's blood, there is no concern for rejection or disease transmission.

PRP therapy is a non-surgical process. The time it takes to draw a patient's blood and process it through an FDA-approved lab kit and then inject it into a patient, takes less than 15 minutes. Despite the placement of injections in sensitive areas, there is no downtime associated with the procedures. Patients have literally gone into their doctor's office during their lunch break, received the injection and returned to work.

PRP Treatment History

In the 1990's, "growth factors" became a buzz word in the medical community and more than 30 years later, it is clear that growth factors play a key role in all kinds of healing. In truth, scientists began looking into using platelet-rich plasma for wound healing as early as the 1970's, but the equipment needed to separate PRP from a patient's blood was expensive enough to prohibit using PRP in common practice (**www.prolotherapy.com**).

As the cost of the equipment lowered in the 1990's, PRP treatments made headlines in sports medicine. High-profile professional athletes successfully received PRP treatments soon translated into wide-spread PRP use in other therapeutic areas. The demand and availability for smaller machines grew, so it became possible for physicians to create PRP treatments from small samples of patient blood right in their office, as I do in my practice.

In the 2000's, PRP branched into more and more areas of medicine. It eventually caught the attention of physicians who wanted to provide their patients with a more "natural" solution for cosmetic repair. That's when Dr. Charles Runels — the eventual developer of the O-Shot™ and Priapus Shot™ — began his work with PRP.

"I began using PRP for the Vampire Facelift™, and then later, the Vampire Breast-lift™," Dr. Runels explained. "I was working with my female patients on nutrition and weight loss and found that once they reached a certain point, they wanted to quit because their facial skin started to sag."

"Since using PRP for a facelift is a simple, non-surgical procedure, I decided to add it to my practice and encouraged my patients to 'treat' themselves for their weight loss achievements," said Dr. Runels. "This rejuvenated their skin *and* spirits so they continued with the fitness and nutrition objectives."

Dr. Runels wrote about the events that led to his development of the O-Shot™ in his book *Activate the Female Orgasm System: The Story of the O-Shot*, published in 2013. Since he administered the first O-Shot™, together we have trained hundreds of providers worldwide in the procedure. It is important for me to emphasize that as much as I champion these procedures, receiving PRP treatments from a certified doctor with FDA-approved PRP medical devices of the highest quality is imperative for treatment success.

Dr. Runels made it his passion to train doctors specifically on administering the O-Shot™. Like many of my colleagues, I was already using PRP for the Vampire Facelift™ when I heard Dr. Runels speak about incorporating PRP into treatments for sexual wellness. I cannot describe how clear it was that this would be revolutionary for treating sexual disorders and urinary incontinence. I knew immediately that I was going to dedicate myself to practice, promote and train others.

It was in March of 2012 when Dr. Runels invited me to join him in training physicians around the world on the Vampire™ series of aesthetic treatments, as well as the O-shot™ and Priapus Shot™.

Together, in July 2014, we successfully published the first ever academic paper on the use of PRP for female sexual dysfunction in the Journal of Sexual Medicine. This is a landmark paper as it brought to light the effectiveness of the O-shot™ and has stimulated interest in the study of PRP for the treatment of Lichen Sclerosis and Vulvodynia.

PRP as a Preventative Strategy

I have seen platelet-rich plasma treatments produce tremendous results in terms of restorative benefits for both sexual wellness and treatment of incontinence. However, I believe PRP also has great potential as a preventative strategy to hold off these conditions altogether. By using the patient's own blood to create PRP, and by harnessing the body's own healing power, tissue can regenerate and potentially stave off degenerating and aging effects.

Since PRP therapy can be used for tissue rejuvenation, to preserve muscle tone, tissue sensitivity, and blood flow, it can actually help to prevent problems that cause sexual dysfunction and incontinence. Even more exciting than solving embarrassing medical concerns is the promise of avoiding them altogether.

Whether PRP therapy is used as a proactive or reactive measure, it has tremendous promise for creating total sexual health in men and women of all ages. Please be sure to read the patient testimonials from those who want to share the wonderful benefits from PRP therapy.

Is PRP Treatment Safe?

The medical research for PRP shows no side effects when the shots are prepared with an FDA approved kit. The FDA has approved approximately 20 different lab kits for this purpose. The reason the procedure is so safe — regardless of the medical specialty administering the procedure — is because the platelet rich plasma is taken from the individual's body and therefore considered autologous. There are no foreign bodies to which the person can have a reaction. As previously mentioned, PRP has been used in multiple lines of medicines and it has proven safe in all instances.

In the specific use of the O-Shot™ and Priapus Shot™, it's commonly wondered if there is pain associated with having a needle inserted in one of the most sensitive bodily regions. Topical numbing agents are used in the area where the needle is inserted; patients experience little-to-no pain during the injection and little-to-no soreness later.

The safe, non-surgical, out-patient and pain-free aspects of the treatment make it a very desirable procedure when faced with other, more pervasive options.

Why Chose PRP Therapy If You Are Already Receiving Other Treatments?

If you are already receiving hormone treatments or on prescription medication for sexual dysfunction, you might wonder what's the added benefit of PRP. Later in this book, I will detail when PRP is combined with other treatment options it produces optimal results. For now, I'll outline the advantages of using PRP; it's not just a short-term solution to problems.

Outside of bio-identical hormone replacement, most strategies that address sexual dysfunction only deal with treating the symptoms and not the curing the problem. PRP therapy offers a Regenerative Medicine approach to a solution for sexual dysfunction. You might need to receive more than one injection over the course of time, but PRP works to correct many of the issues *behind* sexual dysfunction, such as damaged or desensitized nerves or compromised blood flow and gland function.

Because PRP therapy is sourced from your own blood and leveraging your body's ability to heal, you are essentially helping yourself correct years of damage from the effects of aging in a way that medications and other procedures simply cannot address. The O-Shot™ or the Priapus Shot™ is a progressive way for your body to achieve a younger, more sexual you.

The science behind this process is being used to enhance sexual functions for men and women of all ages. By stimulating blood vessel growth and nerve regeneration, men can experience improvements in their erections while women report greater sexual arousal.

Why opt for chemical symptom treatment of sexual dysfunction when the path to sexual joy might lay best in self-healing? The O-Shot™ for women and Priapus Shot™ for men are injectable PRP treatments designed to heal the individual's tissues and organs.

The treatment rejuvenates the orgasm system by stimulating stem cells found in the tissue and by delivering activated growth factors to the desired site. New blood vessels and sensory cells are formed and work to increase function and improve sensitivity. The entire injection procedure takes less than five minutes and requires no patient downtime. My patients typically experience improved function within a week and report improvements in sensitivity, heightened arousal and enhanced sexual function over the next 10-12 weeks.

When compared to gels, creams or oral drug treatments, PRP therapy might seem cost prohibitive or more complicated than simply taking a pill. You might be surprised to learn that the expense of oral drug treatments over time will actually be greater than PRP therapy and even combined treatments.

Additionally, PRP offers a freedom that other measures do not — the ability to make love spontaneously.

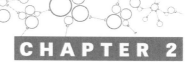

CHAPTER 2

For Women Only:
The O-Shot™

Since Platelet-Rich Plasma (PRP) therapy has proven successful in growing and healing tissue in numerous areas of medicine, using PRP treatments to improve blood flow and sensitivity for women experiencing sexual dysfunction was a natural advancement in medicine. But the journey to what is likely the best breakthrough in treating female sexual dysfunction was not a direct path, to say the least.

Prior to inventing and patenting the O-Shot™, Dr. Charles Runels used PRP for three cosmetic procedures called the Vampire Facelift™, Vampire Facial™, and Vampire Breast Lift™. Multiple news reports described these innovations in beauty treatments. The Vampire™ process has been documented and reported on by the New York Times, Dr. Oz, the Doctors' Show and hundreds of local news stations all over the world.

In these non-surgical cosmetic procedures, the patient's blood is used to create a gel-like substance (platelet rich fibrin matrix, or

PRFM) which is then injected into the desired area of treatment. PRP then goes to work over the next 12 weeks to rejuvenate or "anti-age" the skin. Collagen and elastin are regenerated, improved blood flow and a youthful glow are experienced by most. The skin often clears of acne, wrinkles improve and texture and quality improve noticeably within a few weeks.

When the Vampire Breast lift™ is used appropriately, it can help to enhance cleavage and restore shape to an aging breast. The nipple is often affected post breast enhancement or reduction surgery and it is common to experience diminished nipple sensitivity. PRP can be used to restore sensitivity to the nipple post-surgery. It can also be used to reduce the appearance of surgical scars.

Dr. Runels incorporated the Vampire procedures into his practice and was recommending them as an alternative option to cosmetic surgery. During this time, his girlfriend requested that he adjust the procedure to use in her vagina. In his book, "Activate the Female Orgasm System: The Story of the O-Shot," Dr. Runels tells the story that she made the request to see if the PRP treatment could do for her vagina what she had experienced in her breasts — heightened sensitivity.

Dr. Runels reported that the results of this one attempt included heightened arousal, improved orgasms that were more easily attained and an increase in vaginally-produced orgasms with intercourse. Additional treatments to other patients produced similar results -and often a resolution to urinary incontinence. With such positive outcomes, and no negative side-effects, Dr.

Runels quickly began to offer the procedure to his entire practice and train other doctors, as well.

"I found literally thousands of research papers on the subject of PRP and no serious or adverse side effects were reported," says Dr. Runels.

I first saw Dr. Runels speak about PRP and the Vampire Facelift™ in a conference in Las Vegas a few years ago. As a functional medicine physician, I love employing 'outside-of-the-box' thinking, so when he presented on the regenerative mechanism of PRP, the light bulb went on.

The idea of using your own body to heal and rejuvenate itself was profound. One of the tenets of Osteopathy is that the body has an inherent ability to heal itself. Regenerative medicine is the process of regenerating health and potential. My Osteopathic training prepared me to fully understand the potential benefits of PRP technology.

After the lecture, I immediately invested time and money and was committed to offer PRP procedures in my practice. I began with the Vampire Facelift™, which fit well since I have robust aesthetic artistry practice. While administering the Vampire Facelift™, I began to really see the regenerative benefits of PRP and its potential use in other areas of medicine. By then, Dr. Runels was working with the O-Shot™ and Priapus Shot™. It was easy to see how the procedures could help my patients with sexual wellness and incontinence. I spent some time learning from Dr. Runels and quickly partnered with him to spread the word and train other physicians in the use of PRP.

Dr. Runels described how his female patients in their 60's, who were hormonally correct, received the O-Shot™ and reported having the best orgasms of their lives. My patients share similar experiences — some of which you will read about in later chapters. In addition to improving sexual wellness, I have seen women with varying levels of urinary incontinence achieve healing through the O-Shot™. I do not know if I can tell you which group of women is happier with their results!

To date, we have each trained and certified hundreds of doctors from around the world who now offer these procedures. Though I was among one of the first physicians certified by Dr. Runels, it has been a privilege to not just offer the Vampire™ series of aesthetic procedures and the O-Shot™ and Priapus Shot™ to my patients, but to also train many other physicians in these sought after procedures.

Some women might want to stop reading and sign up for the treatment. 'Finally,' you might be thinking, 'a female answer to Viagra!' I can understand your excitement, but the O-Shot™ is so much more. And for those of you who are not yet convinced, keep reading for more information about the science behind this life changing procedure.

The Best Shot You Will Ever Get

Research shows that 30 to 50 percent of women report conditions ranging from sexual dissatisfaction to sexual dysfunction. With 150 million women in the US, (2010 Census) the low end of this statistical range means 50 million women suffer from sexual problems. The exciting news about PRP treatment (or the O-Shot™) is that it can help these 50 million women experience sexual pleasure that they might have given up on achieving.

When Dr. Runels first administered what became known as the O-Shot™, he did not just inject the vagina; he also injected the clitoris. This might sound painful, but I have found that in my practice the application of a powerful numbing gel eliminates most, if not all, discomfort a woman feels with this procedure.

The process of naming and trademarking a product is lengthy and complex, but the O-Shot™ (or Orgasm Shot™) received its name because of the long (and short-term) effect Dr. Runels noted in his earliest patients. The rejuvenating benefits of the O-Shot™ (or PRP therapy) is often seen quickly, but it takes up to 12 weeks to be fully realized. There is histology (study of tissue) evidence that the regenerative power of PRP is still at work at 10 weeks after injection. This means that reversal of the tissue aging process is still working at 10+ weeks.

Dr. Runels reports that many patients received an immediate benefit from the shot and several of his patients became highly sensitive (even hyper-sensitive) to clitoral orgasms within hours after the procedure.

If a woman experiences this type of immediate sensitivity due to the impact of the PRP on the clitoris, the sensation usually fades pretty quickly. However, the healing benefit of the PRP leads to more frequent and stronger orgasms, increased lubrication, and other desired effects. The placement of the PRP when doing the O-Shot™ is vital to the success of the treatment.

"This area appears to be critical in determining whether a woman is able to achieve a vaginal orgasm, something experienced consistently by fewer than twenty percent of women," explained Dr. Runels.

When Dr. Runels first decided on placement, he based it on his understanding of a woman's orgasm system. By injecting PRP in both the periurethral space in the vagina and visible part of the clitoris, tremendous results were achieved in terms of sexual healing. To visualize the placement of these shots, please see Diagram A.

Women who receive the O-Shot™ find that the PRP treatment stimulates stem cells to grow healthier vaginal tissue. My female patients who have struggled with decreased sensitivity, decreased ability to orgasm, vaginal dryness, low sexual desire, and even pain with sex have seen vast improvements in overall sexual function, desire, and performance with the O-Shot™. Benefits women report include:

- Greater arousal from clitoral stimulation
- Younger, smoother skin around the lips of the vagina
- A tighter vaginal opening
- Strong and more frequent orgasms

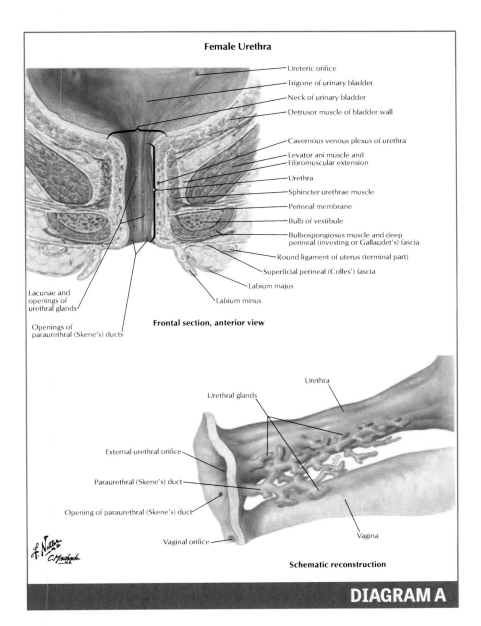

Female Urethra

Ureteric orifice

Trigone of urinary bladder

Neck of urinary bladder

Detrusor muscle of bladder wall

Cavernous venous plexus of urethra

Levator ani muscle and
Fibromuscular extension

Urethra

Sphincter urethrae muscle

Perineal membrane

Bulb of vestibule

Bulbospongiosus muscle and deep
perineal (investing or Gallaudet's) fascia

Round ligament of uterus (terminal part)

Superficial perineal (Colles') fascia

Labium majus

Labium minus

Lacunae and
openings of
urethral glands

Frontal section, anterior view

Openings of
paraurethral (Skene's) ducts

Urethra

Urethral glands

External urethral orifice

Paraurethral (Skene's) duct

Opening of paraurethral (Skene's) duct

Vaginal orifice

Vagina

Schematic reconstruction

DIAGRAM A

- Elevated desire for sex
- Improved ability to experience a vaginal orgasm
- Increased natural lubrication and decreased pain during sex

The treatment has proven beneficial for many women in my practice regardless of age or if they are pre or post-menopausal. This treatment should only be administered by a medical professional who is trained and certified. Though my office is one of the leading providers in PRP treatment, it is my prediction that these procedures will quickly become standard of care. I will continue to qualify more physicians in hopes to improve access to the O-shot™ and Priapus shot™ for men and women around the world.

How Long Does it Take to Work?

PRP is injected into the periurethral area of the vagina and the part of the clitoris that is externally visible. (See Diagram A.) PRP is injected just behind the clitoris and is absorbed in the corpora cavernosa (internally attached to the clitoris and can be several inches in length).

When Dr. Runels injected PRP into his first female patient, he noted that the fluid traveled into the corpora cavernosa (Runels 2013). In his experience, and mine, the results of this can be an immediate effect of hyper-sensitivity and extreme sexual desire. Many women who have received the O-shot™ have reported an intense desire to masturbate later that day, a feeling which can continue for several hours.

This condition may be a direct result of the PRP treatment at work as the regenerative activity of the activated PRP creates significant metabolic activity and an immediate increase in blood flow to the area. We have captured this activity using an ultrasound that measures blood flow. The hyper-sensitivity does not happen for all patients. It tends to wear off relatively quickly. In addition to the increased blood flow to the area, it is likely related to the volume of PRP causing pressure on the women's urethra. In a subsequent chapter, I will explain the close relation between the urethra and a woman's sexual system. This relationship is pivotal to understanding why the O-Shot™ helps with both sexual healing and stress incontinence.

It actually takes two to three weeks for the PRP treatment to begin rejuvenating cells and tissue growth. We find this to be true in all PRP therapies. After that time, the vast majority of patients begin reporting healing symptoms to a wide-array of sexual dysfunction concerns. These include an end to painful intercourse, increased desire, vaginal lubrication and intense orgasms. In fact, many women report having the best orgasms of their lives — and some of these are post-menopausal women in their 60's!

PRP therapy provides both rejuvenation and healing to people in various areas of medicine. In some instances, a patient may only need a single treatment. In other cases, on-going PRP therapy is needed to maintain positive results. The healing that occurs because of PRP treatment never reverses, but since the body continuously ages, one treatment is not permanent.

Depending on the level of healing that your body needs, one shot may provide rejuvenation that will last for months or even years. If you start to realize the benefits from the O-Shot™ begin to subside, a second shot might eventually be in order. However, I would say most of my patients are still experiencing the benefits of their first O-Shot™.

Side-Effects that Rock!

The primary purpose for the O-Shot™ is to regenerate the vaginal tissue and clitoris; however, there are some remarkable possible side effects. Patients can experience any of the following:

- An instantly jump started arousal
- A cure to urinary incontinence
- Improved sleep patterns
- Mood enhancements
- An increased desire to exercise, lose weight, and live better
- Improved relationships

The instant improvement in libido can be caused from the hyper-sensitive stimulation to the clitoris that some women experience. Though it can be an intense experience for women and their partners, it does lessen with time as the long-term improvements to sexual wellness become more evident.

A cure for urinary incontinence is incredible, yet was unintended from the O-Shot™. However, it is explainable. In the female body, the urethra exits between the clitoris and vagina (See Diagram

B). The muscles and nerves in a woman's body that control the urethra and bladder also impact vaginal functions. The close proximity of these systems in relationship to each other means that weakness in one region can impact its neighbor. This is why pelvic floor disorders effect sexual and urinary health.

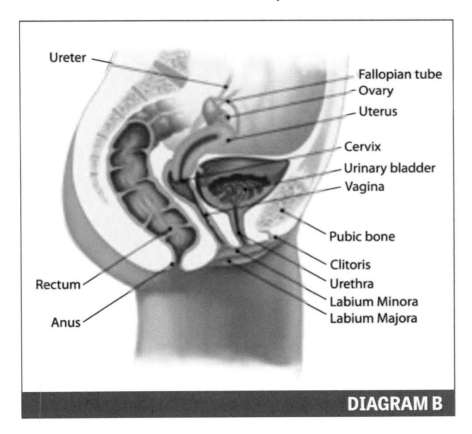

Ureter

Fallopian tube
Ovary
Uterus

Cervix
Urinary bladder
Vagina

Pubic bone

Clitoris
Rectum
Urethra
Labium Minora
Anus
Labium Majora

DIAGRAM B

Besides increased arousal and a solution to urinary incontinence, many of my patients report improvements to other areas of their lives, including enhanced sleep, better moods, exercise and healthy living. I believe this all comes from reversing the negative effects of sexual dysfunction which can include depression and feelings of unattractiveness. Once sex becomes easier and more enjoyable for a woman, her self-image improves; the desire to eat well and take better care of herself increases.

Additionally, if a woman can experience relief when it comes to urinary incontinence, she is more likely to engage in social and physical activities that may have avoided for obvious reasons.

Finally, the best long-term effect of the O-Shot™ is improved relationships; for both partners. Healthy and satisfying sexual function is a key to a healthy and happy relationship. Of course, a great relationship is developed over time and includes many dynamics; however, intimacy is a relationship glue should never be discounted.

Improving sexual function and resolving urinary incontinence increases self-confidence and ultimately, the quality of life. It's the best thing I could ever prescribe for an individual or relationship!

What the O-Shot is NOT

My colleague who patented the O-Shot™ told me that despite his extensive work with women, he is often perceived negatively for "trying to stick women with a needle in their private parts." Therefore, I thought I should dedicate a little bit of time to go over what the O-Shot™ is not.

The O-Shot™ is not painful. As I have mentioned previously, PRP therapy is used in a great number of medical practices, from hair restoration to wound treatment. While you probably cannot think of a more sensitive area than a man's penis or a woman's vagina/ clitoris, the numbing cream used still renders the procedure painless, as the women in this chapter will attest.

The O-Shot™ is not genital mutation. While I cannot think of too many subjects more disturbing than female castration, the O-Shot™ bears no resemblance to this procedure. The O-Shot™ does not remove or damage a woman's clitoris in anyway; in fact, it is meant to heal and make a woman more sensitive and responsive.

The O-Shot™ is not done for meaningless reasons. I recently heard a famous celebrity tease a talk show host about how men have performance issues as they age and woman do not. For many, many women, that simply is not true. And for many women, hormone therapy is not sufficient to restore what time and age has taken from them. The reality is that a woman's body can "break" sexually; the good news is that there are treatments available, and the O-Shot™ is a big win.

When to Seek Treatment

In my practice, women do not usually seek treatment for sexual dysfunction. In fact, the issue typically comes up as a side note in discussions regarding hormone balance and other health concerns. When prompted, my patients will often admit experiencing changes in their sexual desire and activity, but they do not necessarily want it treated. When I am able to convince my female patients to seek treatment, or when we use the O-Shot™ to address incontinence, they always come back with positive feedback.

I repeatedly hear things like, "I forgot how much I enjoy this," or "I did not realize how much I missed this part of me."

Women are undeniably sexual creatures, every bit as much as men, and they should not only engage in sex, but enjoy it as well. The O-Shot™ has the ability to help women in all stages of life and at various degrees of sexual dysfunction to regain their existence as sexual beings.

The benefits from the O-Shot™ may last long-term or may diminish after a year or two, depending on the original level of dysfunction and how much cellular regrowth is required.

But this procedure has positive impact on self-esteem, confidence, and relationship health that has no shelf-life.

A post-menopausal woman may easily see how *now* is the right time to seek PRP treatment. Yet, a woman does not have to wait until she goes through the "change of life" to want to better her sexual experience.

Pregnancy and childbirth are hard on woman's body and multiple pregnancies can do a combined damage. If childbirth — or other vaginal trauma — has resulted in a decrease in sexual pleasure, there is no reason for a woman in her 20's, 30's, or 40's not to seek PRP treatment.

Since PRP therapy is based on your body and triggers healing and regenerative factors in your system, you will only benefit from seeking that healing earlier in life rather than later. There is no risk; there is no reason a young woman should not use PRP as a preventative measure or an early stop-gap to ensure she never reaches a point of pain or extreme incontinence.

When Dr. Runels first started administering the O-Shot™ he did not begin with post-menopausal women in the 60's. He recounts the story of treating a relatively young hairdresser who had recently had a baby, but whose marriage was disintegrating right before her eyes.

"She experienced structural damage due to giving birth to a very large baby. She was unable to have sex with her husband because of the pain and her marriage was falling apart — they were at the point of filing for divorce," Dr. Runels explains.

"The O-Shot™ restored her system and made it so she could have sex again. She and her husband are now back together and share an intimate relationship. That's the power of the O-Shot™ — to restore relationships and make lives better." Runels said.

Women of all ages may have reasons for seeking this procedure. My patients' needs are wildly diverse from the woman with severe incontinence — desperate to get her life back — to the woman with the insensitive clitoris who had no idea what she was missing prior to PRP therapy. Here are their stories:

Testimonials from Women

T. A. who came to the office for help during menopause

"There came a time in my life when I was feeling lost, out of control, lonely, sad, crazy, and all alone. I did not want to talk with anyone, not even my husband. Something was going on within me that I had never felt and I was unsure of what it was. My libido was next to nothing and I was having severe hot flashes that resulted in severe headaches. After plenty of research I finally figured out I was in menopause.

I tried various remedies to no avail when a good friend told me about Dr. Roy and Doctors Studio. I went to her website which was the best decision of my life.

My husband and I met with Dr. Roy who spent over an hour with us going over my tests, answering questions and offering suggestions. Among my hormonal treatments were pellets — a combination of testosterone and estrogen.

However, the pellets did nothing for my libido. I discussed more options with Dr. Roy and eventually decided to get the 'O Shot™.'

AMAZING!!!! It has totally worked for me. It took approximately two weeks for it to kick in, but really kicked in about two months after the shot. I have been on the upside ever since. I would totally recommend it to anyone as it has been a great experience.

My sexual desire is back and there is definitely no dryness; I finally feel like a woman again. If the day comes and the 'O Shot™' wears out, I will definitely be the first one to sign up for another one. For ladies that are worried about pain, it does not hurt!!!"

Susan who came to me for help with menopausal symptoms

"I had been feeling down, no energy, and experiencing stomach problems. I did some research on my symptoms and was sure I was going through menopause. I started looking into hormone replacement therapy and found Dr. Roy. She was so nice and sweet and said, 'I can help you in more ways than one.'

She went over several things with me, including diet, (bioidentical) hormone replacement therapy, etc. She discovered that I was born without a clitoris, which is pretty important for a woman. I was married and had children, but somehow this was never identified. I had surgery on my urethra, and it should have been caught then, but it wasn't.

We discussed having surgery to expose the clitoris. I had an O-Shot™ before the surgery and had feelings in that area for the first time in my life. After the surgery to expose the clitoris, I had a second shot.

I'm in my 50's and finally feel like 'Oh, this is what everyone is talking about.' Prior to treatment, I did not even know what it (orgasm) was supposed to feel like! Dr. Roy has basically opened up a whole new world for me.

People might wonder how this can happen, but in my day, we did not talk about this kind of thing. Even now it's bizarre to talk about, but I would not want anyone else to go through what I went through — which includes a bad marriage, divorce, and a bad sex life for years.

The O-Shot™ is not painful and it is worth the benefits. I feel like a 50-some-year-old virgin in many ways. I understand my body now better than ever before. Dr. Roy is so sweet and very reassuring. She told me, 'I will help you, and you will have an orgasm.' She has the drive to want to help people, and that is why I love her so much!"

Suzanne who was experiencing problems with incontinence

"Dr. Roy was recommended to me for aesthetics. Whenever I walked into the office for treatments, it became a little bit of a joke because I always had to run to the bathroom. During one appointment, I told Dr. Roy about my recent diagnosis of a bladder issue. I had just gone through a treatment but with no relief.

Dr. Roy told me about the O-Shot™ and how besides helping with sexual function, it has helped some women with incontinence issues. I had the shot, and within the first couple of days, I could go a little longer without rushing to the bathroom. It kept getting longer between bathroom visits. Then, I noticed I was exercising and was not having any urinary leakage.

Of course, I also got one of the most amazing benefits from the procedure as well. I had no trouble reaching climax before the shot, but my orgasms intensified, and I had them more often.

At one point, I was considering having a second shot, but I spent time using the Apex device Dr. Roy gave me to help with Kegel exercises. I thought I was doing a proper Kegel, but the Apex really made a difference. After using that for a while, I never needed a second treatment.

You know, my husband used to cringe when I would go to a doctor, because he knew a bill was coming, but with Dr. Roy, there are no complaints. My husband saw a benefit, as well. And really, it was a huge benefit for my whole family! It let me get back to a normal life — that's what Dr. Roy has given me."

Cheryl who was experiencing problems with incontinence

"When I met Dr. Roy three years ago, I was in pretty bad shape. All the results from my blood work were off. Now, everything is right in line without any need for medication. This was accomplished completely through nutritional changes.

While working with Dr. Roy, I started bioidentical hormone treatments. This made a great difference. I also received the Vampire Facelift™ and O-Shot™.

I had the O-Shot™ procedure one time and it changed everything. It brought everything back in a good way. Prior to the shot, sex was actually painful. The pain stopped, and sex was enjoyable again. I also went from no real interest to a very active sex drive. I absolutely recommend the shot for others, because it makes a huge difference."

O.D. who decided to augment hormone treatment with PRP therapy

"A couple of years ago, I did some Internet research on bio-identical hormones and met Dr. Roy. Later, I became interested in other anti-aging procedures she offered. Afterward, I decided to try the O-Shot™. I followed up with a second shot about six months later.

It has been a very interesting experience for me and I recommend it to everyone. When I hear women describe their symptoms, I tell them they need to try to O-Shot™. It has been more worth it to me than any cosmetic or augmentation procedure I've had to date.

Sexually, I experience a better response, improved lubrication, faster and longer and more impactful climax. In fact, I was never the kind of woman who experienced female ejaculation and now I do. All in all, it is a better experience than I've had — even in my twenties.

The whole procedure was completed quickly — it took maybe 35 to 40 minutes from the time my blood was drawn to the injection. It was pain free and I never had any discomfort; even after the numbing cream wore off. In fact, I was sensitive for a while, but in a good way. That sensitivity lessoned a little over time, but the experience was still very good.

Intercourse was much more pleasurable and exciting."

C. C. who was having minor stress incontinence issues

"I was seeing Dr. Roy for aesthetic treatments and went to an open house for the Vampire Facelift™ and saw very positive results. My face was bright and people commented how great I looked. My skin appeared warm and bright, and I was often asked how I kept myself looking so good.

At a later visit, the subject of the O-Shot™ came up because I was experiencing the "sneeze and pee" incontinence. I decided to give it a try and it worked great — I do not have any more issues with incontinence.

It has been a very positive experience for me and it did not hurt at all. It was a simple procedure that I hope more doctors start offering so more women can benefit from the results."

M. R. who wanted to deal with issues of incontinence and insensitivity

"I started seeing Dr. Roy for hormone imbalance and some incontinence issues. I began with a hormone treatment and she told me about the O-Shot™, which I went ahead and did.

At this point, she's balanced my hormones. Also, I had to wear underwear guards and I don't have to do that anymore. What is great about Dr. Roy is her thorough testing and questionnaire and how she spends so much time to identify your issues and possible solutions."

S. B. who needed to address dermatological and health issues

"I started seeing Dr. Roy because I was dealing with a rash and sinus headaches and after going to two dermatologists without getting results, I thought a holistic approach would be best. I did some work with Dr. Roy on diet and my issues cleared up. While working with her, I filled out her questionnaire and identified some other issues she could help me with such as incontinence and painful sex.

I have had the O-Shot™ twice and I think the first one really did the trick. My incontinence issues have significantly improved and I can have sex again and enjoy it.

Other doctors I saw would just shrug or act like I did not say anything when I talked to them about sex being painful. I am amazed at how women's issues like this are not more heavily considered. I would recommend the treatment to anyone; it is amazingly helpful."

R.V. who first received PRP treatment for aesthetic reasons

"I've worked with Dr. Roy a great deal and think what I found most significant was the PRP treatment on my face. I had really dark circles under my eyes because of family history and allergies. Dr. Roy just put a little PRP treatment around my eyes and lips — not even a full Vampire Facelift™ — and it made a big difference.

When my son came home from college, he said to me, 'Mom, your skin looks so great.' I think it was a big compliment that he could see such a difference. But at the same time, I did not look like I had cosmetic work done. People would just say, 'Oh, did you get a haircut' or 'Are you wearing new makeup' so they could see the difference, but they could not put their finger on what was done.

I didn't really think I needed the O-Shot™ at that time — I just volunteered to be part of a training for Dr. Roy. However, I still noticed a big change and so has my boyfriend. It was painless and very non-traumatic and I saw a difference pretty quick. Orgasms are definitely stronger than before.

I think it's great that you can have small things done that really add up to major results; especially instead of going through surgery."

CHAPTER 3
For Men Only: The Priapus Shot

Platelet-Rich Plasma (PRP) therapy has proven successful in growing and healing tissue in numerous areas of medicine. Using PRP treatments to improve penile blood flow and sensitivity is a natural advancement in medicine.

The process of using PRP to help with sexual dysfunction is based on the idea that a man's inability to achieve or maintain and erection or reach orgasm is due — at least in part — from problems with blood flow, loss of sensitivity and tissue damage. These are exactly the symptoms that PRP therapy improves. The development of the Priapus Shot™ is a revolutionary idea that Sherlock Holmes would call, "elementary."

Possible benefits men can receive from the Priapus Shot™ include:

- Improved firmness of erection
- Enhanced blood flow and circulation in the penis/pelvic area (making it easier to get an erection)

- Greater sensation in the penis head (making it easier to achieve orgasm)
- Elevated sexual pleasure and stamina

Men can experience sexual dysfunction for many reasons; medications, decrease levels of testosterone, enlarge prostate. PRP stimulates tissue growth and rejuvenation in the penile tissues, thus improving erectile and sexual potential.

Why a Shot Instead of a Pill?

Since men have solid options for oral treatments like Viagra and Cialis, the thought of having something injected into their penis might seem absurd and downright petrifying. Certainly many of my colleagues, including Dr. Runels who patented the Priapus Shot™, tend to promote the O-Shot™ more in their practices.

Perhaps it's because men seem to have other options available between oral medications and testosterone treatments. Dr. Runels himself has said he wants to place his focus on the O-Shot™, because women have so few options for sexual healing.

While I can understand this point of view, I've found men in my practice who could not benefit from oral medications. Healing through PRP therapy has worked. One of the most encouraging results of the Priapus Shot™ is that men who have experienced nerve or tissue damage due to surgery or diabetes have shown amazing regenerative results.

Most importantly, **I advocate PRP therapy for men because it is healing at the tissue level, and therefore, will help to either preserve function or to contribute potential for rehabilitation of erectile function. PRP seems to make all other treatment options work better.**

My approach is to use all the tools available to facilitate optimal sexual function. Physicians can't build a house with a hammer alone, nor can the body reverse the consequences of aging with just one pill. Now, put a pill together with Priapus Shot™ and you have synergy.

If a man can have his sexual function improve then his sexual activities are no longer dependent on timing, scheduling, or planning ahead. It's obvious our culture has an impact on a man's ability to achieve an erection, the size of his erection, and other related objectives. This has a large impact on his self-confidence and self-esteem. An oral medication might be able to help a man have sex, but it cannot restore the intangibles that come from a properly working sexual system. The Priapus Shot™ can help return a man's spontaneity and confidence.

I believe it is vitally important for men and women to experience sexual wholeness and wellness as they age. PRP offers men the opportunity to achieve wellness by regenerating the sexual organ and therefore, regenerating sexual potential.

How Can Getting a Shot in My Penis Be Good?

As one of my patients puts it later in this book, 'the thought of having a needle in your penis can be petrifying.' As a woman, I wouldn't know, but I can sympathize; I've had to do a bit of reassuring with my female patients injecting a needle in their sensitive areas as well. For men, I can assure them that the needle is small and a numbing agent prevents pain and significant discomfort.

Injecting medications into the penis to restore function is not a new concept. In fact, prior to the development of oral medications, injectable procedures were one of the most prominent treatments for sexual problems. If you think there's no way you would have a shot in your penis, please keep reading about the potential upside. And as you do, keep in mind that my patients also report zero downtime associated with the treatment. Men continue with their normal activities and can even engage in sex immediately following the procedure.

While there are other treatments you can seek for erectile dysfunction, none of them have the rejuvenating and regenerative benefits of PRP. If you are seeking long-lasting heightened sexual function and joy, the PRP treatment is truly a positive development for you to consider. The art of treating sexual dysfunction is in the combination of treatment modalities. In my opinion, all strategies should include PRP.

How Long Does it Take to Work?
How Long Does it Last?

Like other PRP targeted treatments, a period of two or three weeks is required for a man to fully realize the results of the shot. How long the results last will vary for each patient, but I recommend a regimen that involves two to three treatments in the first year and then annually thereafter.

The protocol for the Priapus Shot™ requires the use of a penile pump post injection. This is recommended so that the PRP is moved throughout the penis and more tissue can benefit from the healing triggers of PRP therapy. It might seem awkward to use a pump on your penis, but it is important to distribute the PRP gel throughout the tissue.

While men have seen benefits of PRP without the pumping exercise, proper use of the penile pump can help achieve the ultimate results faster and longer.

While multiple treatments may be needed for some men to receive optimal benefit, over the course of a year the cost turns out to be less than that of oral treatments. **That means a man can regain his sexual spontaneity and flexibility with just two or three short doctor visits a year.**

Men can start losing testosterone in their 30's. As many as forty percent of men in their 40's report some kind of sexual dysfunction. That number increases to seventy percent for men in the 70's. While that is a staggering percent for older men, you can see that even young and middle-aged men might have reason to seek PRP therapy.

When Dr. Runels finally broke into treating men with PRP, his first patient was a younger man looking to improve his sexual performance for his soon-to-be-bride.

"I had been performing the Vampire Facelift™ for several months when I received a call from a young man. He was a conservative man of faith and had not yet had sex with his fiancé. His marriage was in a month, and he wanted help enhance his penis," Dr. Runels explained.

"His size had been an issue for him. I knew PRP could improve blood flow so it might prove beneficial with penile girth. I proposed a treatment plan and made it known that it was only a theory, not a proven science. My patient decided to proceed with what I came to call the Priapus Shot™.

I spoke with him after his honeymoon and while he did not report growth, he said everything was working so much better. He had harder and more frequent erections and was pleased with the results," Runels said.

So, as you can see, PRP therapy is not just an "old man's game." Men might find reason to seek treatment as a preventative measure or to recapture some part of their youthful vigor even if they are still fully functional.

Testimonials from Men

Anonymous (Name withheld at Patient Request)

"I have an ongoing interest in evolutionary biology, so part of my motivation to receive the Priapus Shot™ was for the science. I have a willingness to be a guinea pig where I do not see much downside or risk -which was the case in receiving the procedure.

I was taking an oral medication that had negative sexual side-effects. PRP treatment was something that I thought could help. The result of the PRP treatment was positive, even though it diminished over time.

I have had three shots now in a little over a year and I will continue the process as I do see the benefits. I would also recommend it to others."

Anonymous (Name withheld at Patient Request)

"I came to know Dr. Roy while receiving hormone therapy from her partner. I did not need to correct any sexual dysfunction because I was having great success with the testosterone treatments, but I thought I would see how the Priapus Shot™ could help.

To date, I have had three shots with Dr. Roy and still receive testosterone treatments every week. My experience has definitely led to increased sensitivity. As with any rejuvenating treatment, I think the skin feels smoother and there is a more youthful appearance.

My wife received the O-Shot™ at the same time as my first treatment. We felt it was well worth the investment; I definitely recommend the treatment to men.

I admit there was a little fear factor involved with having a needle in my penis and I think if most men hear that, they would say, 'no way'! But contrary to what you might think, it is not a painful experience. You do feel something during the treatment so it can be awkward, but not painful. There is no down time. You can literally have sex the same night."

Anonymous (Name withheld at Patient Request)

"My wife was going through menopause and we were looking into treatment options. That's how we came to know Dr. Roy. My wife began with hormone treatment and eventually got an O-Shot™ and it really worked well for her.

I went through an evaluation and decided to switch from a testosterone shot to pellets per Dr. Roy's recommendation, which ended up working well for me. I originally sought testosterone treatments because of fatigue, but eventually noticed issues with some sexual dysfunction. I have had the Priapus Shot™ twice now and have been very pleased.

After the first treatment I did not try the pump; however, I am pumping regularly with the second shot. The procedure is pain-free and there is no downside to the treatment."

Anonymous (Name withheld at Patient Request)

"I am in my mid-50's and I keep in pretty good shape. I am on hormone therapy and sought Dr. Roy for PRP treatment.

The shot was a painless procedure and I saw quick results. The benefits from the first shot lasted about eight months and I went back for a second treatment when the upsides started to wear off. I did not have any sexual dysfunction issues to start with, but I would say the shot 'turned back the clock.' I experienced more firmness and fullness and increased sensitivity.

It is a natural, non-invasive procedure which is what attracted me. There are no chemicals involved; what is being injected into you is your blood. The treatment was pain-free and quick, which was my biggest concern. The whole procedure lasted 20 minutes. It was a very positive experience and I would do it again."

CHAPTER 4

My Practice & The Patient Experience

My team at Doctors Studio is successful in treating hundreds of men and women for hormone imbalance and sexual dysfunction; specialized expertise in making complex diagnosis and treatment decisions. My top priority is patient dignity and professional integrity. That means results are absolutely the sole focus of our practice: both patient experience and functional change.

We are bioidentical hormone experts, extensively trained in functional, regenerative and anti-aging medicine, and highly skilled in medical artistry. I can hear you asking, "What is medical artistry?" It is the ability to understand complex and expanded mechanisms of action, and then apply a complex multi-variant solution that is focused on results, both functional and aesthetic.

You have heard it said that your body is a temple; I could not agree more. Your body must be well cared for and treasured as a temple should be. But I also believe that "you" are more than just the sum of your parts. Therefore, you must not only be nourished physically, but also mentally, spiritually, and physiologically. While I am treating my patients, I seek to apply medical treatment strategies that impact the essence of their entire being.

In my practice, I help women and men suffering from symptoms and conditions that are more than just age-related challenges or inconveniences. The impact that hormonal imbalance, thyroid disorders, adrenal fatigue, and even incontinence has on a person's life can be extreme and may result in depression and a serious decline in their quality of life. The treatment plans I design involve customized wellness programs that blend personalized nutrition and fitness regiments with natural solutions, such as bioidentical hormone therapy and PRP treatments.

The treatment protocol is an individualized combination of treatment modalities to directly support the various aspects and mechanisms of sexual function: psychogenic, physiologic, habitual, etc. Patients are then treated and monitored with the goal of rehabilitation and improved satisfaction.

Some of the concerns/conditions, I address in my practice include:

- Women experiencing symptoms of menopause
- Men experiencing symptoms of andropause (male menopause)
- Male and Female changes in sexual function and dissatisfaction
- Incontinence: both stress and urge incontinence

The connection between whole body wellness, disease prevention, and functional medicine is made by treating the body according to biochemical and physiologic principles. Instead of treating a host of symptoms, the focus is on treatment strategies on leveraging the body's inherent ability to heal itself; reestablishing balance and wellness with diet, targeted supplements, specific exercises to stimulate hormonal response and with prescription drugs or surgery when necessary. To this end, I blend the following approaches:

- Platelet-Rich Plasma Therapy (Priapus Shot™/O-Shot™)
- Hormone imbalance and bio-identical hormone replacement (BHRT)
- Weight loss and nutritional testing/guidance
- Healthy aging and fitness routines
- Detoxification and optimization of metabolic system

What Men Can Expect

When a man comes into my office for a full evaluation of erectile function, a preliminary work-up is performed and a review of his history and laboratory findings. The patient is asked to complete an extensive symptom questionnaire to help identify underlying causes of the changes and difficulty he is experiencing. A blood draw identifies basic sex hormone levels including testosterone and estrogen. This is a simple screening test used to help determine the need for a more comprehensive hormone evaluation to make sure that hormones are at ideal levels (testosterone is high enough and estrogen is low enough) for a man to be at optimal health.

As part of the physical evaluation, a penile Doppler is used to quantify blood flow within the penis. This test helps determine if the blood flow and function of the penis is optimal or if there are issues that need to be addressed. There is also a biothesiometer used to assess the level of penile sensitivity. When sensitivity is lost, it increases the difficulty for a man to obtain and maintain an erection. Loss of sensitivity is common when a man has diabetes, hormone imbalance, and is also often a part of a normal aging process.

The goal of the evaluation is to better understand the physiology of the problem and to design a treatment strategy that is focused on rehabilitation. The desired outcome is to restore "successful and satisfying sexual function". This notion of "successful and satisfying sexual function" is unique to each man.

The rehabilitation strategy is a combination of interventions that focus on addressing the cause of erectile changes and the improvement of erectile function. A custom formula of technologies is combined to address the individual need of the patient. Some of the tools and technologies that are applied are as follows:

1. Platelet Rich Plasma — a regenerative medicine treatment rejuvenates the sexual organ

2. Testosterone replacement and bio-identical hormone therapy

3. Nutrition and targeted exercise

4. Treatment of underlying condition

5. Oral ED medications

6. ICP: a painless auto-injection of vasodilators that cause the penile tissue to expand

7. Penile pump to stimulate repair, rejuvenation and growth

8. Sex therapy: satisfying sex requires health of mind, body, spirit

A few words about some of the strategies...

Typically, I offer a combination of therapies that include PRP treatment(s), bioidentical hormone therapy, and injectable vasodilator, penile pump, and/or Cialis. Not all of these treatments will be necessary long-term, but working collectively they stand the best chance of restoring full functionality, improving erectile function and sexual wellness.

Not all of my clients have the same goal for PRP therapy. Some might use it to prevent degeneration while others use it for regeneration once a change in function has occurred. For example, one patient had a single PRP treatment and was then able to use oral medication to achieve erections consistently. Another has had three Priapus Shots™ in the last nine months and feels an enhanced function with each subsequent treatment. And yet another man had a decrease in sensitivity after a penile injury that was partially restored with the first Priapus Shot™.

The Doppler evaluation helps in creating an injectable cocktail that will generate an erection for select/desired period of time. This erection will last regardless of stimulation or climax and can be an effective way to help restore penile function for men experiencing sexual dysfunction; both erectile dysfunction and premature ejaculation.

If you are wondering why I might recommend that a man use an injectable to trigger an erection, I have to refer you to what we know about the penis. Simply put, the penis is a "use it or lose it" body part. Lack of use or stimulation can lead to the penis becoming fibrotic and it often loses both strength and size. Conversely, the robust erection that is safely achieved with a custom formula ICP can initiate cellular changes and functional improvements when done at least three times per week, but no more than every 24 hours.

The regenerative powers of PRP with the rehabilitative success of ICP is a synergistic combination that often facilitates a full restoration of successful and satisfying sexual function.

There are many ways to combine the technologies to accommodate lifestyle, cost and comfort level. The success of sexual rehabilitation largely is determined by the scope of the problem, the way the tools are combined and the quality of the education provided to the patient. The patient will leave my practice with full understanding of treatment protocol and use and emergency instructions.

Proper follow up is necessary to dial in maximum rehabilitation potential. Additional PRP injections may prove to be helpful.

What Women Can Expect

Like men, women are evaluated for hormone imbalance and other causes of decreased libido and changes in sexual function. Quite often, women have changes in their sexual experience due to hormonal shifts that happen during childbirth and menopause. It's common to develop a lack of interest or vaginal discomfort, dryness, and/or a change in sensitivity and arousal.

I evaluate the general health of my patients and design protocols to restore balance to the complex female sexual system. Patients complete a comprehensive survey and the symptoms of urinary incontinence is explored in depth. Understanding the physiology of the problem leads to more effective treatment design.

The rehabilitation strategy is a combination of interventions that focus on addressing the cause of sexual changes and the improvement of sexual desire and function. A custom formula of these technologies is combined to address the individual need of the patient. Some of the tools and technologies that are applied to this include:

1. Platelet Rich Plasma — a regenerative medicine treatment rejuvenates the sexual organ

2. Estrogen/Testosterone replacement and bio-identical hormone therapy

3. Pelvic Exerciser to strengthen orgasm response and improve pelvic bowl health

4. Treatment of underlying condition

5. Compounded medicated creams applied to cause increased blood flow and ease of arousal

6. Bioidentical hormones to restore vaginal tissue integrity

7. Sex therapy: satisfying sex requires a healthy mind, body, and spirit

The O-Shot™ works best when a woman is hormonally balanced. Yet, the O-Shot™ also works quite well as a standalone treatment to improve vaginal sensitivity and lubrication or to help with urge and stress incontinence. If a woman experiences a decline in sexual function after menopause, I usually advocate for a comprehensive hormone evaluation in conjunction with the shot. Balancing hormones is ongoing so evaluation can be done before or after O Shot™.

The area around a woman's urethra contains a network of blood flow and sensory nerves. This "periurethral" area is the target for PRP rejuvenation. This functional target lies along the top wall of the vaginal canal. The clitoris extends from the exterior of the body into the corpora cavernosa and can be several inches in length. Some think that a vaginal orgasm is similar to stimulating the clitoris from the inside of the vagina while others feel that the sensation arises from the bundle of nerves surrounding the urethra. In any case, the procedure works best when the area around the highly sensitive urethra is infiltrated with the rejuvenating power of PRP.

Testosterone hormone plays a key role for women to experience sexual desire and a sense of vitality. Too many women have less than optimal testosterone levels and are suffering from lack of sexual motivation. Restoring testosterone can be done very safely and effectively. Optimal testosterone in women is necessary for bone health, brain health, muscle and metabolism health as well as sexual health.

An electro muscle stimulator or manual muscle contraction device is recommended to improve pelvic muscle tone, strengthen the intensity of the orgasm, and to help restore urinary continence when it is caused by deconditioned pelvic musculature.

The combination of therapies improves sexual function, response and desire. Each treatment modality addresses a physiologic aspect of the female sexual system. A comprehensive approach is often required for optimal results. All protocols include PRP regenerative therapy.

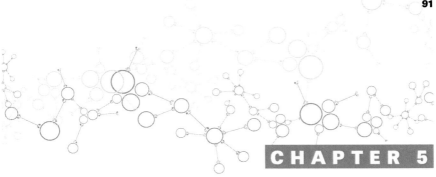

CHAPTER 5

Testimonials from Physicians

Dr. Charles Runels developed the trademark use of PRP in treating sexual dysfunction in men and women several years ago. The development of PRP in medical treatments has been explained, but using it as a tool to treat sexual dysfunction is less than five years old.

While the procedures are perfectly safe and miraculous in results, you may find that your doctor has as much knwowledge of the O-Shot™ and Priapus Shot™ as you do (actually since you are reading this book, you probably know even more).

Medical advancements are not made overnight, but rather based on decades of research. Once breakthroughs do happen, spreading the knowledge to physicians as well as the public takes time — sometimes years. During this time, new therapies are researched, proven, and gain wide-scale acceptance. PRP therapy for sexual dysfunction is still considered cutting-edge medicine.

While I could hardly treat every patient who could benefit from the O-Shot™ and Priapus Shot™, I am dedicated to training other doctors in these procedures. To date, there are several fully trained providers using the procedures in their practices nationwide.

While not many doctors across the United States are using PRP therapy for treating sexual dysfunction, there are several of us who are on the cutting edge in this area of medicine. This section contains comments from my colleagues regarding the reasons and science behind the treatment in their own words and the successes they have seen in their practices.

Colleague Testimonials:

Dr. Hugh Melnick, Advanced Fertility Services, New York, NY

"Having practiced what I believed to be 'cutting edge' medicine for more than 35 years in the fields of reproductive endocrinology and gynecology, I have been involved in treating patients from the very beginning with such miraculous medical therapies as out-patient in vitro fertilization and non-invasive laparoscopic gynecological surgery.

From the day that I first 'hung up my shingle' in 1976 to the present time, women's healthcare has undergone an amazing transformation, yet no adequate therapies have been developed for two of the most common health issues affecting a huge number of women and their quality of life: sexual dysfunction and urinary incontinence.

Although there are existing treatments for these conditions, the surgical, medical and hormonal therapeutic interventions currently available have been far from universally successful in curing many women who suffer with these disturbing problems. There are different types of Female Sexual Dysfunction and Urinary Incontinence, but the most common forms of these two diverse conditions actually have similar features that are at the root of both problems!

The common causative feature is the lack of healthy connective tissues, nerves and blood vessels in the vagina, the urethra and the bladder. When there is inadequate blood flow to the vagina, there is a loss of connective tissue and the outer vaginal tissues become thin, causing dryness. With some of the sensory nerves being too close to the surface of the vagina, due to its thinness, a woman experiences burning and painful intercourse. In addition, without the proper blood circulation, other sensory nerves responsible for erotic and orgasmic sensation, which are found in the area between the vagina and the urethra (where the urine exits), deteriorate and a woman's sexual responsiveness is diminished or lost.

Likewise, when there is not enough connective tissue to support a woman's urethra and bladder and the nerves which normally control bladder function are not functioning properly due to compromised blood circulation in the area, urinary incontinence occurs. Since the loss of connective, nervous and circulatory tissues in an identical anatomic area- the area between the front wall of the vagina and the urethra- is at the root of both conditions, it is not surprising that Platelet Rich Plasma (PRP) injections into that area can be curative for both problems. When a time tested therapy, such as PRP injections, which has proven to be an extremely safe, totally natural and effective treatment in other fields of medicine, was first applied to the treatment of female sexual dysfunction, not only did it relieve a large percentage of women's sexual dysfunction, but was noted to coincidentally cure urinary incontinence in women who were treated for painful intercourse and lack of orgasmic responsiveness. This coincidental scientific observation points out the validity of PRP therapy.

In medicine, there is a long established rule called Occam's Razor, which says that if a common cause of several diverse symptoms (sexual dysfunction and stress urinary incontinence) can be demonstrated by curing both with one therapy, the common and simple explanation is the correct one. In this case, from the clinical responses of women treated thus far with PRP therapy, the common cause of both sexual dysfunction and urinary incontinence, was the absence of key structures — connective tissue, nerves and blood vessels in the vagina, itself, and in the area between the vagina and the urethra. The injection of Platelet Rich Plasma, which has been activated to produce tissue growth factors, cause new connective tissues, nerves and blood vessels to be formed, so that sexual and urinary function becomes clinically improved. Once new blood vessels and connective tissues are regenerated, hormonal therapy becomes more effective, since there is improved vascular circulation to the area, which enhances the effect of estrogen on the vaginal tissue."

Dr. Julian Keiffer, East Valley Naturopathic Doctors, Mesa, AR

"I have been using PRP in an aesthetic sense (the Vampire Facelift™ and Vampire Breast Lift™) for years and lately I have been using it on a surface level with some fantastic results. When I heard Dr. Runels speak about using PRP to treat sexual dysfunction, it was like being hit by a bolt of lightning! I thought, 'I have to do it; there is real promise.'

I was one of the first four doctors to train and use the therapy. I provide many services in my practice so the O-Shot™ and Priapus Shot™ are just two of my tools. I believe the PRP needs to be combined with hormone therapy because when they are, I have found great success.

The interesting change I have seen for women is that the O-Shot™ does not just help with painful intercourse or increased lubrication, but it changes their overall libido. I had one husband say that he feels like he got the 18-year-old version of his wife back.

I think both procedures have the ability to change lives and save marriages. The treatments do not just improve people's sexual wellness, but they improve their overall health and outlook as well."

Dr. Kristen Kalmbacher, Bayside Regenerative Medicine, Fairhope, AL

"I was classmates with Dr. Roy and have been using the O-Shot™ and Priapus Shot™ in my practice for a couple of years. I have had people say that it has been revolutionary for their sex lives.

I think the shots work best when combined with hormonal therapy, so I use a hand and hand approach with hormones and PRP. I would say about thirty percent of my patients are receiving hormone treatments and about five percent of those have used the O-Shot™ or Priapus Shot™. That is a small amount, but I have had really good results with those patients.

I think people who are having painful intercourse or are unable to have orgasms at all, they are top candidates for the procedures. Treating those two conditions are the main reasons I present the treatment option to my patients, and so far, I have had a hundred percent success rate."

Dr. Charles Runels, Fairhope, AL

"I began using PRP treatments in my practice for facelifts. I strongly promote nutrition and healthy living and as my patients began to lose weight, they would reach a point where they wanted to stop because the skin in the face would start to sag. I found PRP cosmetic treatments to be a perfect way to address this concern and my patients felt confident about continuing their weight loss routines.

Eventually, I moved into using PRP to repair or enrich sexual wellness. While I have developed treatments for both men and women, I actively promote the O-Shot™. Part of this is because I have this background of working with women and ninety percent of my patients are women. But also because even without advertising the Priapus Shot™, I still get calls about it.

I find that it is hard for women to discuss sexual concerns of dysfunction with their doctors. Research has proven that even if women talk their doctors about sexual problems that most doctors are not comfortable or knowledgeable on how best to treat them. It seems to me that women do not always get support from other women in this matter either. The idea that a woman's body or vagina specifically cannot be broken is ridiculous. So women deserve to be able to seek treatment and get a treatment that works.

The O-Shot™ is that answer. More than 90 percent of the women in my practice who have received this treatment have seen improvement in their sexuality and resolution of their stress incontinence. Having treated thousands of women in my practice, I believe this success rate demonstrates that PRP can change the lives of many, many women."

Dr. Hayley DeGraff, Advanced Life Clinic, Huntsville, AL

"We started doing PRP treatments at my office about a year and a half ago and we have had great success with the procedure and very high patient satisfaction. Our patients have been pleased with both the comfort of getting the treatment and the results.

We treat men and women who report an inability to achieve orgasm, experience a loss of sensitivity, and other issues associated with aging. We combine the PRP treatment with a focus on addressing hormone changes. We tell them that the procedure is designed to restore a more youthful anatomy.

I believe there is going to be more and more research, study, and use of PRP and the applications will grow. This is just a very exciting point to be in aesthetic medicine."

2

The Importance of being a Sexual Being... and You Thought it was Just for Fun!

In Maslow's hierarchy of needs pyramid (which is pictured in Diagram C), sex is considered part of a human's most basic physiological need along with air, food, drink, shelter, warmth, and sleep. We know very well we can't survive without breathing -and sleep deprivation, warmth, or even shelter can lead to serious illness. But we rarely consider the negative impact sex -or lack thereof- has on our bodies (**www.simplepsychology.org**).

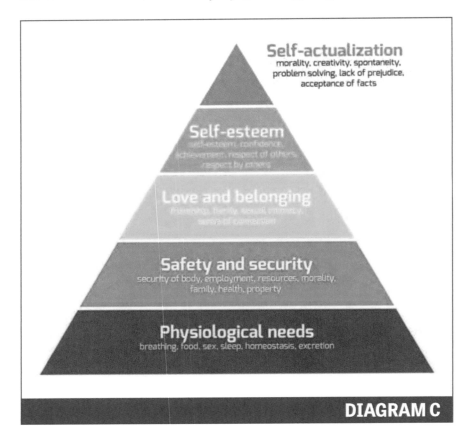

DIAGRAM C

As you can tell by Diagram C, Maslow did not just account for intimacy as a physical need. He incorporated affection, love, and romantic relationships on the third level. According to Maslow, both levels are part of the journey to humans achieving actualization.

I think it comes as little surprise that we are a species fascinated with sex along with the experience and the perceived benefits we receive. As a result, there has been a great deal of research into this subject. According to WebMD, some potential benefits of sex include:

- Stress Release
- An Improved Immune System
- Lower Blood Pressure
- A Source of Exercise
- A Decreased Risk of Heart Attack
- Pain Relief
- Improved Sleep
- Enhanced Mood

How can anyone look at that list and think sex is something we should purposefully deprive ourselves from? But a good sex life seems to correlate to more than just the immediate benefits from orgasm, and the hormones released during and after the experience. The results of extensive research seem to indicate that Maslow might have been right – taking care of the physical need for sex enriches our lives in more advanced pursuits.

As a further demonstration of Maslow's correct understanding of human needs, plenty of research shows that people who have sex four times or more per week also earn higher wages than individuals with less active sex lives (**www.huffingtonpost.com**). The correlation is probably related to any — or all — of the above benefits. What I want you to take away is that **maintaining the vitality of sex will lead to extraordinary relationships and higher quality of life.**

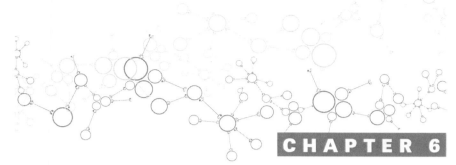

CHAPTER 6

Why Sex is Important Physically

As we learned from Maslow, sex is a physical need. Yes, need. Not desire, not want, not wish — need. For a variety of reasons, we often understate how important sex is in the United States. Oddly enough, we do this while simultaneously selling sexual images throughout our culture.

Visually we know we are sexual beings, but intellectually we tell ourselves we are not slaves to our "animal" instincts. I think it is vital to our health that we eliminate this way of thinking. We also need to dismiss antiquated ideas like, sex is for reproduction and not suitable for "older" people.

Sex is a basic physical and psychological need that does not disappear as we age past our child-bearing years. There are many physical and psychological benefits to the sexual experience, orgasm, and related release of hormones and chemicals. The upsides of sex include stress release, increased immunity, increased health, and even pain relief. So contrary to the old joke that sex might "kill" you, **the truth is that sex can lead to a far healthier you!**

Stress Relief

Sexual activity is often associated with the release of hormones such as oxytocin — "the love hormone" — that have certain positive effects on both men and women. As a result, it is thought that reaching climax during sexual engagement acts as a stress release for both genders.

Besides the release of hormones that improve mood, sex offers better sleep. After an orgasm, a different hormone — prolactin — is released. This hormone is one that is responsible for feelings of relaxation and sleep. For this reason, sex can lead to a nice slumber which allows a person to wake-up feeling rejuvenated and in good spirits.

While this is certainly a positive impact of sexual function, the absence of or difficulty in achieving climax can cause a lot of tension between a couple. Both sexual dysfunction and incontinence can place undue stress or pressure on a relationship, which can amplify the underlying condition.

Successful treatment for sexual dysfunction and incontinence will therefore lower the stress levels of the person experiencing the condition by relieving any worry about being unable to perform or disappoint one's partner. There can also be a noticeable increase in the harmony of the relationship once these conditions are treated.

Regarding urinary incontinence, proper treatment alleviates all stress and allows a woman to experience greater sexual freedom, improved social interaction and independence. Eliminating the ever-persistent worry about going out in public can immediately relieve depression and anxiety.

Immunity

People who have sex at least once or twice a week possess a higher level of defense against germs, viruses, and other harmful pathogens. According to WebMD, an active sex life correlates with people taking fewer sick days from work.

Scientist at Wilkes University in Pennsylvania found a thirty percent increase in antibodies that fight against the cold and flu in individuals who are sexually active a couple of times a week. (**www.prevention.com**).

Increased Health

Sex is good for your health! Men who have sex at least twice a week are fifty percent less likely to die of heart disease than men who rarely engage (**www.webmd.com**). Since there is also a link between sex and lowering blood pressure; the case can be made that a good sex life can lead to a longer, healthier life.

For those of you who are accustomed to counting calories, sex burns about five calories per minute. A fifteen to twenty minute love making session can burn seventy-five to a hundred calories.

Grant it, that's only about half the calories of most candy bars, but sex can be more fun than spending an extra ten minutes on the treadmill.

Pain Relief

Women, if you ever had the "I have a headache" excuse, lean in... research has found that orgasms can block pain because they release a hormone that helps raise your pain threshold. Orgasms have been noted to reduce menstrual cramps, arthritic pain, and yes — even headaches (**www.webmd.com**).

CHAPTER 7

Why Sex is Important Emotionally

The physical benefits of sex are clearly understood, but there's even more to gain. If we go back to Maslow's hierarchy of needs, sexual intimacy is listed at level three. While sex is very good for the body, it is also good for the inner being.

Love and sex are two different things, and a relationship should encompass both. A good sex life enriches intimacy and romantic attachments. On a chemical level, when a man or a woman experience an orgasm, hormones are released in the brain that trigger a desire to attach or "cuddle." This can keep the intimacy between a couple strong over a life-long relationship. Sexual wellness can also improve an individual's mood and outlook on life.

Relationship Impact

When you are in a committed, monogamous relationship and one partner's sexual interests significantly decreases, it is likely going to be cause for concern to the other individual. What differentiates your romantic relationship from all other relationships is the intimacy you share during sex. When something disrupts that shared experience, it is a cause for concern for both individuals.

When romantic partners seek couples counseling, they often face sexual issues of some sort. A decrease in sexual activity might not be the core problem, but it's big red flag. As a result, therapists will seek to engage both members in discussion and attempt to open lines of communication in order to identify what is the deeper cause to the lack of intimacy.

While therapists will address any number of issues a couple may need to work through, they are not qualified to run labs or perform examinations. If the problem is medical or physical, ultimately no amount of counseling can restore intimacy; however, as a rehabilitation it is incredibly helpful and strongly recommended. The therapist can help facilitate the development of patience and support within the relationship and the couple often grows from the experience.

Given the large numbers of individuals who experience some degree of sexual dysfunction at some point in their lives, open communication can help avoid misunderstandings. Without honesty and openness, the person experiencing the sexual issues will probably withdraw their affection. Alternatively, the unaffected partner might continue to try to initiate sex and begin to experience high levels of rejection and hurt.

I cannot stress enough how important it is to talk to both your partner and your doctor when you notice signs of sexual dysfunction or incontinence. Keeping your partner informed might be embarrassing, but it could prevent bitterness and resentment from tearing your relationship apart. Additionally, communication can help maintain intimacy even when sexual activity may decrease.

When considering how important sex is for a couple, please remember there is a biochemical reaction to orgasm for both men and women. Chemicals are released in the mind and body that produce loving and bonding feelings. There is no other natural way to generate these chemical reactions.

Feeling desired or wanted is integral part of a person's self-image, confidence, and mental health. If this is ignored, then it may result in one partner filling their needs outside of the relationship. I personally do not believe most individuals want to cheat on their partners; however, it happens and is in fact, quite common. Yet, my experience tells me that it is not always the individual's first preference.

I have had several men come into my office and tell me that they want to be intimate with their partner, but if that cannot happen, they would consider looking outside the relationship. And men are not alone in their infidelity as we often think is the case. Statistical compilations indicate that more than 50 percent of men and women admit to committing infidelity at some point.

The number decreases between married couples, but 22 percent of men still admit to straying at least once during marriage and 14 percent of women admit the same. What's even more telling is that 74 percent of men and 68 percent of women say that would have an affair if they knew they would never be discovered (**www. statisticbrain.com**).

The difference between individuals cheating on a boyfriend or girlfriend versus their marital partner indicates that couples really do value marriage. But why would people say they would cheat if they could get away with it? I can think of many of reasons — some cynical and some not. My antidotal experience takes me back to sexual wellness and that **all individuals need to feel wanted and desired**. Confidence and self-image are based not just on the intimacy between two people, but also the longing to feel attracted.

Since we spend so much time emphasizing how love and sex are different, my next claim might not be very mainstream. I believe that restoring sexual function between a couple should be the first step in addressing relationship problems, not the last. After years of treating men and women for sexual dysfunction, I am confident that restoring sexual wellness might be enough to bring back the closeness and intimacy between a couple. There's a healing that ensues between two individuals when they are sexually intimate. Once ability is restored then couples can explore other areas of concern, if problems persist.

Family Dynamics

If sexual dysfunction can hurt relationships, then it can negatively impact the family unit. Perhaps when people married earlier in life and started a family, it was less likely that issues such as sexual dysfunction could adversely influence young children. But census data shows that the average age of first time mothers has increased from 21 to 25 over the last several decades and more women are waiting until their 30's to become first-time mothers.

This could very well be a natural outcome from increased life spans, but the point in time when a man or woman experiences sexual dysfunction has a greater chance of occurring while they are still raising children. When parents lose intimacy with each other, it can contribute to marital disharmony, coldness between the couple, infidelity, and divorce.

While it is always sad to see a marriage fail, the impact a divorce has on young or adolescent children compared to grown children is very different. For this reason, addressing the issues of sexual dysfunction early is important for the marriage and family.

The link between sexual dysfunction and depression is well documented. Feelings of attractiveness and desire are so important to an individual's positive self-image that without experiencing sexual climax and the chemicals that are released could aid in depression. Whatever the causal agent behind this link, what matters most is that the link exists. Depressed individuals who are not receiving treatment do not make great lovers or parents.

The typical treatment for depression — anti-depressants — can make matters worse between a couple as several medications are known to impact sexual functions. However, going untreated is not an ideal situation either. Seeking help that addresses the sexual disorder itself — particularly natural solutions — could prove beneficial for sexual and mental health. Of course, the need to talk to a doctor first is crucial in understanding what came first: the chicken or the egg. But if depression issues or lack of self-confidence are developing because of sexual dysfunction, it is very likely that romantic relationships and ultimately family dynamics will become strained.

It can be very difficult to understand depression from the outside looking in and it can be equally difficult to understand the feelings of inadequacy associated with sexual dysfunction. Furthermore, it can be nearly impossible to understand how actions can devastate relationships. Withdrawal, depression, and lack of desire cause painful feelings of rejection and even convince a partner that all love is lost.

Infidelity does not always happen because a person is promiscuous or wants greater sexual variety than their monogamous relationship allows. While love does not equal sex, I have never come across a survey or poll that showed people were happier in sexless marriages. A full commitment to maintaining intimacy while addressing sexual dysfunction can make the difference between a happy family dynamic and a "cold home."

Certainly relationships can survive and even thrive albeit sexless... but if those extraordinary couples were given a choice, most would chose a sex filled marriage.

Children know when someone is amiss in their parent's relationship. They might not be able to identify or articulate the problem, but they can sense when they are not close or intimate. When couples realize their marriage is broken, but elect to stay together "for the children," the children grow up not witnessing a fully functional intimate, loving relationship. This can ultimately do as much harm to the children as a divorce. Ergo, protecting your family is not just about "staying together" it is about staying intimate, achieving total health, and living well.

If you are experiencing sexual dysfunction and just cannot bring yourself to discuss it with your partner, please seek medical attention to correct the issue as soon as possible. Divorce rates are far too high to allow something that is easily correctable to erode a loving relationship and damage the family unit.

Confidence/Self Esteem

Sexual dysfunction and incontinence can destroy an individual's confidence and self-esteem. If a person does not seek the advice of their doctor and get medical treatment, the hit to their confidence can lead to bigger problems.

In regards to sexual dysfunction, if a man or woman is experiencing discomfort or difficulty in their sexual activity, the person might become less likely to try to participate. As a result, the issues of sexual dysfunction can transform from physical or pharmaceutical to include psychological obstacles as well.

While open communications with your partner (and an understanding partner) will help, not everyone will feel comfortable being open to such a discussion. In those instances, addressing the problem with your doctor should at least facilitate faster treatment and solutions that will minimize the condition.

In regards to incontinence, the condition can lead to a complete lack of desire to engage in sexual activity or any other physical activity that has been known to trigger incontinence. Fear of embarrassment is a natural hindrance to self-confidence and it can lead to avoiding social settings and physical activities. Once a person begins to avoid social activities, the potential for low self-esteem and even depression significantly increases.

Exercise, healthy choices, and complete sexual wellness are keys to enjoying life at any age. Deliberate physical activity, a good diet, and healthy choices such as limiting alcohol consumption and tobacco use can all increase sexual abilities. Additional treatments such as natural hormone therapy and/or PRP therapy might also be useful in enhancing sexual experiences. Once full sexual wellness is achieved, self-confidence and general happiness will dramatically improve.

I have witnessed this hundreds of times in my practice and assure you the same will be true for you.

Quality of Life

As discussed above, a couple that maintains a healthy sexual and intimate relationship has a positive influence over their marriage and family. This projects the quality of their life. Being able to perform sexually (even with assistance) can also improve psychological wellness and a person's overall outlook.

When Viagra went to market in 1998, the idea that it was "ok" for middle-aged couples to want to maintain an active sex life, despite whatever obstacles they encountered, seemed like a revolutionary concept. Then again, the oldest group of Baby Boomers — the generation of Woodstock and "free love" — just entered their 50's. It is little wonder why over the next decade oral medications prescribed to treat erectile dysfunction became a multibillion-dollar industry.

The generation that would not "trust anyone over 30" and women who burned their bras demanding sexual equality, were not willing to give up their sex lives as they aged. Marketing initiatives that drove this multibillion-dollar industry, led the campaign to 'maintain a high quality of life into the golden years'. While some people conjure ideas of old men in nursing homes getting erections that they don't know what to do with, the truth is that a much younger crowd will benefit from treatments for sexual disorders.

We can more easily recognize that stress and urge incontinence have a negative effect on the quality of life (the correlation between nursing home admission and incontinence is actually well documented), but more people accept this condition as something aging individuals (women in particular) just have to accept. This simply is not true. Furthermore, since the correlation between depression and incontinence is well established in women, it is important to understand that solving this problem will improve their general outlook and quality of life significantly.

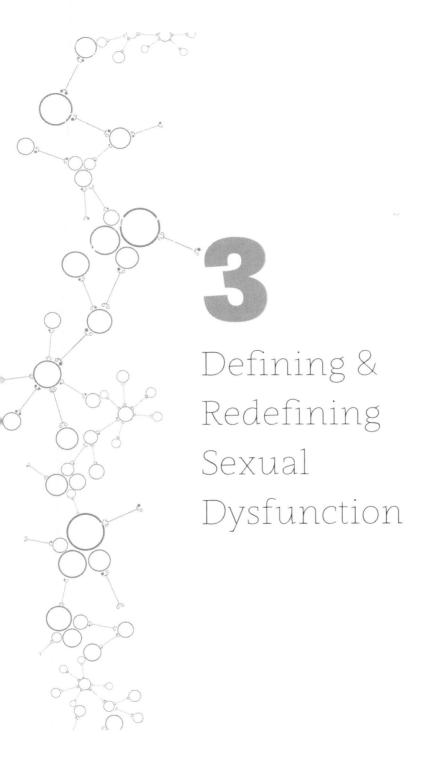

3

Defining & Redefining Sexual Dysfunction

While sexual dysfunction is not life threatening to men or women, it is still important to seek treatment and achieve full sexual wellness. However, since sexual disorders carry varying stigmas and levels of embarrassment, many individuals never seek treatment. They conclude they can just "live with" these conditions and that it is a part of "growing old." Again, I want to assure all my readers that this simply is NOT true!

The first — and most important — reason for discussing your sexual health with your doctor is that sexual dysfunction is often a harbinger or symptom of a larger medical problem. If you are experiencing any of the signs or symptoms already mentioned in this book (or ones described in subsequent chapters), you should schedule an appointment with your healthcare provider. But aside from sexual dysfunction being a potential sign of other larger issues, it is important to seek treatment for other reasons as well.

Sexual dysfunction impacts women and men in different ways. Generally speaking, sexual dysfunction refers to any issues that arise during the four phases of the sexual response cycle that prevents the individual from experiencing a satisfactory sexual experience. This means that any issue that prevents or arises during excitement, plateau, orgasm, and resolution stages constitutes a problem.

For my practice, I cast a far wider net than most medical professionals because I define sexual dysfunction as "any change of sexual function that leaves the individual or their partner felling less than satisfied with their sexual experience."

Less than satisfied might not mean incapable of having sex, but just not happy with their own sexual performance — both physical and psychological. For instance, many men are able to perform sexually, but they find it increasingly difficult with time and subsequently develop anxiety around sexual performance. This can become serious enough that they start avoiding sex or that their anxiety actually complicates the physical demands necessary for a confident engagement.

This is just one example of how sexual dysfunction is truly a degenerative condition — both physically and psychologically. Part three of this book is dedicated to defining — and hopefully redefining — sexual dysfunction. I want you to understand how the female and male sexual system is supposed to work and how it can break down in subtle ways, over time, leading to significant decline in quality of life.

These chapters focus on defining the problems of sexual dysfunction for men and women in broad terms. Of course, many people with these conditions already know that something is wrong. However, they might not be able to correctly identify the exact problem they are experiencing. For this reason — and issues related to embarrassment — men, and especially women, will often not seek help. The problem of sexual dysfunction is far more expansive than most realize.

50 percent of men and women report sexual dysfunction severe enough to interfere with their lives.

So, if you are experiencing difficulty in sexual performance, you are very clearly not alone. Please note that the statistic is that of men and women who say their sexual issues interfere with their lives. Many more never discuss sexual decline or concerns with their doctors.

Unfortunately, this trend of underreporting creates a gap between diagnosis and treatment. The percentage of people dealing with some form of sexual dissatisfaction could be higher than we can accurately estimate. Therefore, half the population might not properly represent the number of people who experience a decline in sexual function and satisfaction.

Some people do not think this is a big deal. Some have been living with sexual dissatisfaction for years and see no reason to address it as a medical condition. I want to change that way of thinking by educating you on the physical, psychological, social, and spiritual benefits of healthy sexual function!

It's important to remember that men and women of all ages deserve to have a pleasurable and confident sexual experience. This is not something you need to sacrifice just because you are growing older. The symptom of sexual decline should never be ignored. If you need a reminder to how your system is supposed to work and what it looks like when things go wrong, continue reading.

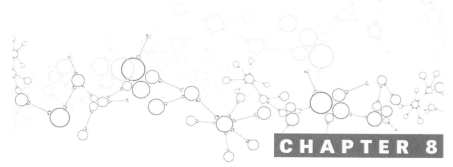

CHAPTER 8

How the Female Sexual System Works & How it Can Breakdown

If you became sexually aware after 1981 when the term "G-spot" was coined in a Journal of Sex Research article titled "Female ejaculation: a case study," then you might be more aware about female orgasms than your predecessors. It might even surprise you that women were not always thought capable of having orgasms. But the fact remains the female orgasm can be elusive, and figuring out if it's because a woman has a sexual disorder — or other issues — can be complicated.

By contrast, the male orgasm is not particularly elusive. Many adolescent boys experience their first orgasms without really trying. Long before a teenage male engages in oral sex or intercourse, he has likely experienced several orgasms through masturbation or wet dreams.

Conversely, research suggests that **as many as 15 percent of women report having never experienced an orgasm at all** — at any age. For those women able to achieve the elusive orgasm, research suggests that seventy-five percent of all women cannot reach orgasm through intercourse alone. These women need extra stimulation to help them climax (James 2009).

If a woman is not open to clitoral stimulation for societal or religious reasons, then it can be difficult for her to enjoy sex and she might not even think she is supposed to. These are the constraints that young women face as they come into sexual maturity and as a result, women often experience their first sexual climax after they lose their virginity, sometimes years later.

Debate still rages whether or not the G-spot is real. In some studies, ultrasounds have been used to find evidence of the G-spot in women who report having orgasms during vaginal intercourse (Gravuba 2008). But since so many women report not being able to experience climax this way, it is difficult to tell if the reason the G-spot is hard to find by of lack of experience or some other issue.

Improved lubrication and vaginal sensitivity might help some women increase their ability to achieve orgasm through vaginal stimulation. But since most women who are able to climax need clitoral stimulation, it is important that the clitoris not become desensitized for her to enjoy sex at peak heights. Either way, an inability to climax does not automatically make a woman think she is experiencing sexual dysfunction.

When thinking of sexual relations strictly in terms of procreation, science might even support this lack of concern. After all, women do not need to be strongly aroused or climax during sexual activity to become pregnant. On the other hand, a man's erection and orgasm is necessary for procreation since this is the process by which the man ejaculates his sperm into the women.

If a woman's climax is "unnecessary" how can she know if she is "normal" or if she needs treatment? Can a woman be sexually satisfied without climaxing at all or irregularly? While many women report enjoying sex without orgasm, **surveys report that 33 to 50 percent of women wish they could climax more often (http:// themarriagebed.com**).

For a woman to enjoy full sexual wellness, she must first come to expect pleasure and fulfillment during her sexual experiences, this often includes climax. A woman needs to identify if her lack of orgasm is a lack of knowledge (being able to masturbate and achieve climax on her own for example), the result of an inexperienced partner, or a physical challenge that may benefit from a physiologic solution.

An honest conversation with your gynecologist and/or sexual partner is a good place to begin. Perhaps the use of sexual toys or lubricants or self-education through masturbation can get you started in figuring out if sexual dissatisfaction you're experiencing is something that requires medical assistance or not.

The woman who has never climaxed and desires to do so may benefit from working with a sex therapist so that she can learn more about her body and the way she responds. Once she has started this work it will be easier for her to communicate with her doctors.

There are several conditions that can lead to sexual dysfunction in a woman that have nothing to do with lack of experience or finding the right position. The contents of this book might help you figure out if you should seek medical treatment or not. If you suspect you might have a sexual disorder, seek treatment. Some conditions are more serious than others and your sexual dysfunction could be a symptom of a larger problem.

Before we figure out if you have a sexual disorder, we should discuss how the female orgasm system works and what sex "can" be like for a woman.

How the Female Orgasm System Works

Like pretty much everything else we do, orgasms begin in the brain. The brain receives and sends signals throughout your body and these signals include triggers for sexual stimulation and climax. But it is important to recognize just how the brain engages in the sexual experience.

Research shows as a woman reaches orgasm the left hemisphere of the brain deactivates and she becomes less aware of her environment. A woman literally has to be taken out of her surroundings to relax, release and enjoy herself during sex. Knowing this alone might be the first step in changing your sexual experience for the better!

Turning the brain off during the early stages of foreplay allows blood to travel to the vagina and clitoris. This often produces a warm rush. At the same time, the walls of the vagina start to secrete beads of lubrication that eventually get larger and increase flow.

As a woman prepares for the sexual experience, she becomes more sensitive to stimulation in multiple areas of her body, including the clitoris, anus, and vaginal wall. These areas are in close proximity to each other and connected by muscles, tissues, and blood vessels. The thickness of her periurethral space has been shown to correlate to the intensity of her orgasm. One of the many areas where the O-Shot™ can improve a woman's sexual experience is thickening this region by encouraging new growth and blood flow.

As pre-sexual activity continues, blood continues to flood the pelvic area. Breathing speeds up, heart rate increases, and nipples can erect. The lower part of the vagina narrows in order to grip the penis while the upper part expands to provide room for thrusts.

Eventually, a large amount of nerve and muscle tension builds up in a woman's genitals, pelvis, buttocks, and thighs until her body involuntarily releases all the tension at once; a series of intensely pleasurable waves overtakes her body.

Scientifically, the orgasm hits when the uterus, vagina, and anus contract simultaneously at 0.8 second intervals. A woman can experience between 3 and 15 of these contractions or waves of pleasure. Neurologically, studies have found that areas involving fear and emotion are deactivated during a woman's orgasm.

A woman can experience orgasm through clitoral stimulation or vaginal intercourse. The G-spot which was mentioned earlier is thought to be the driving force behind vaginal orgasms. The location of the G-spot is reported as being two to three inches inside the vagina, on the front wall. Some scientists hypothesized recently that the G-spot is actually a vaginal extension of the clitoris that is more present in some women than in others (Kilchevsky 2012). The researchers concluded that while evidence is lacking for a distinct anatomical site to the G-spot, reports and anecdotal evidence suggest a highly sensitive area in the vaginal wall is certain. If the G-spot is related to the clitoris, the fact that some women find it more easily than others could be a matter of anatomical differences rather than sexual dysfunctions. It is therefore important to remember that women do not need to achieve sexual climax through vaginal stimulation — it is just important that she can orgasm.

Typically, after orgasm, a woman's body enters a state of satisfied relaxation. Other physiological changes include the hypothalamus releasing extra oxytocin into a woman's system, which can be correlated with the urge to bond, be affectionate, and protect. Other hormones released during climax include dopamine (a pleasure chemical) and DHEA, a hormone that boosts the immune system, promotes bone growth, and maintains healthy skin.

How it Can all Break Down

Sexual dysfunction in women is not an easy thing to define — certainly not as simple as it can be in men. If a man experiences difficulty in becoming or maintaining erection or difficulty to climax, he is relatively certain that he is experiencing some kind of sexual dysfunction. On the other hand, a woman's consistent inability to become aroused or climax can be the result of any number of issues:

- **Psychological:** She just cannot clear her head from thinking about work or the kids or her to-do list
- **Stress:** She is just unable to relax enough to get in the mood
- **Experience:** She or her partner lack the experience to bring her to climax
- **Knowledge:** She lacks the understanding of her own body to help her reach orgasm
- **Emotional:** She is feeling sadness or other emotions that prevent her from enjoying sex
- **Relationship:** She does not feel valued as a sexual partner
- **Physical:** She experiences a decline in physical response such as lubrication and engorgement. She may have thinning vaginal walls that lead to a decrease of sexual sensitivity and often she may even experience pain. The sexual organs can be affected by health changes and the change in hormonal balance. She may even lack desire and motivation for sex due to physiologic changes that can be corrected.

Most of these issues fall into the sphere of treatment that is provided by a psychologist, therapist, couples counselor or even a sex therapist. Often the non-physical challenges can be effectively resolved with proper time, commitment, and effort.

There are physical as well as psychological reasons why a woman may be unable to have a satisfying sex life.

I want women to know that complete sexual wellness is a very healthy thing to achieve!

Are you experiencing sexual dysfunction? I like to think of sexual dysfunction in very broad terms. If you are experiencing an issue where you or your partner is not satisfied during sex, then I encourage you to seek help. If you are not quite sure... take the Quiz:

Sexual Dysfunction Quiz for Women

- Do you have extremely low or non-existent interest in sex?
- Is sex painful?
- Do you have difficulty achieving sufficient vaginal lubrication to make sex enjoyable?
- Are you having problems achieving arousal?
- Once aroused, are you unable to remain interested in sex?
- Are you unable to reach orgasm on a regular basis?
- Are you experiencing a decrease in sensitivity in either your vagina or clitoris?
- Have you experienced urinary incontinence during sex?

- Have you experienced light bleeding during or after intercourse unrelated to your period?

- Is your sexual experience unsatisfactory for you or your partner?

If you answered yes to any of the above questions, you should talk to your doctor about the possibility that you have a sexual disorder. To diagnose female sexual dysfunction, a doctor will usually begin by conducting a physical exam and evaluation of symptoms. A pelvic exam and Pap smear are common tests to help evaluate vaginal health. An analysis of attitude regarding sex as well as contributing factors such as fear, anxiety, past trauma, relationship problems, or substance use can help a doctor properly understand the problem and thus recommend a treatment strategy.

This strategy can be multifaceted since the problem can be a combination of the mind, body, and spirit. Bio-identical hormone replacement, diet changes, PRP procedure (O Shot™), counseling, or a combination of many effective treatments may be offered to rehabilitate the sexual response. It is important to understand and treat all aspects involved.

Female sexual disorders have been broken down into several categories. For some of these to be considered a disorder or dysfunction, they must cause the women distress. Others are automatically causes for concerns. I seek to treat any condition that causes a woman sexual dysfunction, but please read on to identify possible causes for sexual dissatisfaction:

Painful Intercourse/Pelvic Pain

Pain is a significant cause for concern, but women are often used to "managing their pain" as they put the needs of family, work, and others above their own medical well-being. Additionally, it can be easy to dismiss pain as a cramp or the onset of a menstrual cycle. But if pelvic pain persists (whether or not you can manage it with over-the-counter medications), it is a symptom to be taken seriously. Pelvic pain in women refers to discomfort in the lowest part of the abdomen and pelvis. Chronic pelvic pain is discomfort in the area below the bellybutton and between the hips that lasts six months or longer.

Pain that occurs during or apart from sexual activity can be the results of several conditions, including endometriosis, a pelvic mass, ovarian cysts, vaginitis, poor lubrication, scar tissue, or an STD. It is important to discuss any discomfort with your doctor.

Pelvic pain can present itself as severe and steady, regardless of activity. Pain that comes and goes intermittently during intercourse, a dull ache, sharpness, cramping, pressure, or heaviness deep in the pelvis all require attention. Pain can be particularly intense during intercourse, bowel movements, urination, or when sitting for long periods of time.

Treatments will vary depending on the ultimate diagnosis. Possible causes include:

Endometriosis

Endometriosis is a painful disorder in which tissue that normally lines the inside the uterus grows outside the uterus. It most commonly involves the ovaries, bowel, or pelvis tissue lining (**www.mayoclinic.com**).

When this condition occurs, displaced endometrial tissue continues to thicken, break down, and bleed with each menstrual cycle. The problem is that this tissue has no way to exit a women's body as typical uterine tissue would during her period; the tissue/bleeding becomes trapped. If endometriosis involves a woman's ovaries, she can develop cysts and scar tissue.

Aside from discomfort and even severe pain, this condition can also affect fertility. If you are experiencing pain in your pelvic area during sex or otherwise, simple tests can diagnose or rule out this condition.

Vaginismus

Vaginismus is a condition where there is involuntary tightness of the vagina during attempted intercourse that can cause discomfort, burning, pain, penetration problems, or a complete inability to have sex (**www.vaginismus.com**).

This condition arises when a woman experiences involuntary muscle spasms or contractions surrounding the vagina. In some instances, it can be so serious that women cannot even use tampons or complete pelvic exams.

Whether this condition is something a woman is experience prior to enjoying intercourse or is a recent onset condition, treatment is available. According to MedlinePlus (a service of the US National Library of Medicine and National Institutes of Health), treatments involve education and pelvic floor muscle contraction and relaxation such as Kegel exercises. Botox injections have been shown to be effective as it weakens the muscle spasms and often break the reflex cycle that develops over time.

Ovarian Remnant Syndrome

Ovarian remnant syndrome (ORS) occurs if any ovarian tissue is left after the surgical removal of the uterus, ovaries, and fallopian tubes (hysterectomy). If any piece of ovary remains in the woman's body, she could develop painful cysts.

Dr. John F. Steege, Professor of Obstetrics and Gynecology at the University of North Carolina reports that endometriosis, pelvic inflammatory disease, and previous abdominal or pelvic surgeries can increase the risk of incomplete ovarian removal (**www. healthywomen.org**).

If you have had a hysterectomy and are experiencing pelvic pain, discomfort during intercourse or painful urination and bowel movements, you should consult your doctor to see if an ultrasound or CT test should be scheduled.

Fibroids

Uterine fibroids are noncancerous uterine growths that may cause pressure or a feeling of heaviness in the lower abdomen. These rarely cause sharp pain unless they become deprived of blood supply and begin to die/degenerate.

The condition develops when a single cell divides repeatedly to create a firm, rubbery mass distinguishable from nearby tissue. Some fibroids go through growth spurts while some shrink on their own. Women can develop fibroids during pregnancy that disappear after birth (**www.mayoclinic.com**).

In some cases, the presence of the fibroids is enough to cause pelvic pressure or pain, which can be magnified during sex. Seek treatment if pain consistently presents itself during intercourse or if you develop pelvic pain that just does not recede. Bio-identical hormone replacement (BHRT) can often be helpful in relieving fibroid discomfort by balancing the hormone signals that stimulate fibroid growth and activity.

Irritable Bowel Syndrome

Irritable Bowel Syndrome (IBS) is a disorder that affects the large intestine/colon. Symptoms associated with this condition include bloating, constipation, and diarrhea. While IBS is treatable, if not addressed, all of these symptoms can be a source of uncomfortable pelvic pain and pressure and thus cause discomfort during sexual intercourse.

Interstitial Cystitis

Also known as Painful Bladder Syndrome, this condition is associated with chronic inflammation of the bladder and the frequent need to urinate. According to the National Kidney and Urologic Diseases Information Clearinghouse (NKUDIC), symptoms of this condition include an urgent and/or frequent need to urinate, pain as the bladder fills with urine or empties, and pain during vaginal intercourse.

Causes of IC/PBS are not easily defined, so treatments are aimed at relieving symptoms. For many women, symptoms disappear with a change in diet. For others, symptoms disappear for a while, but resurface at a later point in time (months or even years later). There are pharmacologic and nutritional strategies that I employ in my clinic that are very successful in resolving the discomfort of interstitial cystitis. I have successfully treated women with O-Shot™ who experience urinary urge as a result of the chronic inflammation.

Pelvic Congestion Syndrome

According to the Society of Interventional Radiology, one third of all women will experience chronic pelvic pain during their lifetime. Pelvic pain can be due to enlarged, varicose-type veins around the uterus and ovaries.

For diagnosis of pelvic pain, a woman can expect a pelvic exam to search for infection or abnormal growths, cultures to identify diseases such as Chlamydia or gonorrhea, an ultrasound or other imagine tests such as X-rays, CTs, or MRIs, and/or a laparoscopy where a small incision is made in the abdomen to insert a camera which gives the doctor a view of pelvic organs.

Medicines from pain relievers to hormone treatments to antibiotics might be appropriate for the above conditions as well as several therapeutic strategies. These include physical therapy, neurostimulation, surgery, and trigger point injections. Finding the cause is the focus of diagnosis which leads to treatment.

Vaginal Dryness

When a woman cannot become physically aroused during sexual activity, this often results in insufficient vaginal lubrication that can make intercourse painful. This situation can be the result of anxiety, inadequate stimulation or a lack of physical factors that are necessary to produce lubrication such as vaginal wall atrophy, Skene's glands degeneration, hormone imbalance, and decreased blood flow to the vaginal wall.

As a side note, if you are unfamiliar with the Skene's glands, they make a fluid that contains some of the same chemical components that come from a man's prostate. These glands can be found near the opening of the urethra, which are outlined in Diagram A.

The glands are associated with female ejaculation and excrete a fluid that is similar to that which comes from a man's prostate. Therefore, if these glands degenerate, the potential for a woman to achieve optimal sexual fulfillment is limited. Of course, the more commonly known factors such as vaginal wall damage and hormone imbalance are vital to vaginal lubrication, but so are these little known glands.

Vaginal dryness is a common occurrence for women during and after menopause though it can occur at any age. It is often a sign of vaginal atrophy or thinning/inflammation of the vaginal walls due to a decline of estrogen and testosterone.

When a woman becomes sexually aroused, the blood flow to her pelvic organs increase and there is an increase in vaginal fluid. As hormone levels change with menstrual cycles, aging, menopause, childbirth, and breast feeding, the consistency and amount of this moisture can change.

Vaginal dryness can be accompanied by (or related to) itching or stinging around the vaginal opening, burning, soreness, pain or light bleeding during intercourse, urinary frequency, or recurrent urinary tract infections.

While there are lubricants that can help with this condition, other treatments that target the cause are most helpful. I use a combination approach often employing multi-faceted strategies such as, Testosterone Pellet Therapy, BHRT creams that contain Estriol, testosterone, and/or DHEA to nourish the vaginal tissues as well as Platelet Rich Plasma (O-Shot™) to regenerate vaginal tissue will restore blood flow, improve sensitivity, and regenerate the Skene's glands that are responsible for vaginal fluid.

Decreased Sensitivity

For many women, vaginal stimulation is not enough to achieve orgasm. In fact, roughly two-thirds of women report only being able to achieve sexual climax through clitoral stimulation. Therefore, a decrease in sensitivity in either area can cause sexual dysfunction.

Lowering the sensitivity in women include vibrators or other items that can damage the nerves around the clitoris. Birth control medications have also been associated with G-spot or clitoral insensitivity (**www.herballove.com**). Researchers are also looking into how blood flow issues can affect the vagina and clitoris.

There are several approaches to increasing clitoral stimulation and improving blood circulation to the genitals, engorging the clitoris, vaginal, and G-spot as well as improving overall sensitivity. Topical vasodilators can help. Taking time to full arousal is essential. I find that Platelet Rich Plasma (O-Shot™) can do wonders for improving sensitivity in this area, thus improving her experience and ability, intensity and ease of orgasm.

Inability to Orgasm

Female orgasmic disorder (FOD) is the persistent or recurrent inability for women to climax. Even when a woman can become aroused and appropriately lubricated, she can still have difficulty experiencing sexual release. In addition to physical barriers, there are several factors that can contribute to this condition, including lack of knowledge and experience or anxiety and stress.

According to the Encyclopedia of Mental Disorders (**www.mind-disorders.com**), to receive a diagnosis of FOD, a woman's inability to orgasm must not come from physiological problems alone or be a symptom of an underlying medical condition. Instead, it is diagnosed when a combination of physiologic and psychological concerns preside.

For classic FOD, treatments can involve psychotherapy and guided sexual exercises. Successful treatment does not mean women will achieve orgasm during every sexual experience, but it will ensure some increased level of sexual satisfaction. PRP can be used to improve physical and physiologic sexual potential as an adjunct to psychotherapy.

However, when a woman becomes unable to orgasm or if reaching climax is simply more difficult than previously, often physical or physiologic changes are the likely culprits. These changes can include medications that interfere with sexual function, hormonal imbalances, atrophy of the vaginal tissues, and degeneration of the sexual system. This is common in perimenopause and postmenopausal diagnosis.

Most women who have previously enjoyed orgasm and sexual satisfaction can be restored to complete sexual function by addressing the cause(s) of their symptoms. BHRT plus Platelet Rich Plasma (O-Shot™) are incredibly effective in these women. Strengthening the pelvic bowl muscles is always part of a comprehensive rehabilitation protocol.

Lack of Sexual Desire

The American Medical Association has estimated that several million US women suffer from what doctors now call "female sexual arousal disorder" (FSAD). Complete or serious loss of interest in sexual activity in women could come from any number of causes. This condition could be the result of hormonal changes, medical conditions and treatments (such as cancer and chemotherapy), depression, pregnancy, stress, and/or fatigue.

If a woman is bothered by low or decreased sex drive, she might be able to treat her own condition through lifestyle changes and sexual techniques. There are also medicines and treatments that prove promising on this front.

When we have a healthy relationship and make time for sexual intimacy, but desire still remains low, it is likely a lack of optimal hormonal balance. I safely and successfully treat women of all ages with Testosterone Pellet Therapy as part of a comprehensive BHRT hormone balancing strategy when appropriate to restore hormonal balance and sexual desire.

There are many health benefits to optimizing hormones. Brain, bones, heart, muscles, mood, metabolism, and sexual system simply work better when hormone levels are optimal. Platelet Rich Plasma (O-Shot™) can also help to regenerate sexual desire since there is a change in tissue response and potential plus a stimulation of the regenerative process.

CHAPTER 9

Why Erectile Function is Subject to Even Minor Cellular Imbalances and What Can Go Wrong

The average man has about 11 erections per day and several each night (**www.sexhealthmatters.org**). Of course, these erections do not always happen because a man is sexually aroused. A man could wake up with an erection or have one due to some kind of reflex or the need to urinate. When a man experiences erectile dysfunction or other sexual disorders, these frequent erections could come to an end.

Since the male sexual experience typically begins with physical stimulation of the penis to achieve erection, loss of ability to achieve an easy erection can be alarming to men. While it is possible for some men to achieve orgasm by stimulating the prostate, function of the penis is still involved. The defining feature of the male orgasm is of course ejaculation — however, some men can achieve orgasm without ejaculation, but there is still some feeling of "release."

The entire male sexual experience involves stimulation in multiple parts of the body, blood flow through the pelvic area and penis, and several nerves in the penis. Sexual dysfunction can come as a result of chemical imbalances that throw off blood flow, damage to tissue or cells around the penis, and several other minor physical factors. Even though the male erection/orgasm seems simplistic, it can be interrupted with the slightest of ease.

How the Male Erection/Orgasm Works

The traditional view of the male orgasm is that there are two stages: emission following orgasm and a refractory period. During sexual stimulation, the accessory organs contract and men can feel the onset of ejaculation. Within two of three seconds, ejaculation occurs, which cannot constrain, delay, or be controlled.

A technique that is effective in increasing a man's stamina is resisting ejaculation. When accomplished, tension builds up and leads to firmer erection and wildly improved stamina. Perfecting this technique takes practice, but the benefits are well worth the time and energy.

The length of a man's orgasm has been estimated to last 10-15 seconds. During the experience, rapid contractions of the anal sphincter, prostate, and penis muscles occur. Sperm is transmitted up the vas deferens from the testicles into the prostate gland and through the seminal vesicles to produce semen.

Except for dry orgasms, the contraction of the sphincter and prostate forces semen to be expelled from the man's penis's urethral opening. As a man ages, the amount of semen he ejaculates tends to diminish as does the duration of his orgasm. With proper hormone replacement, ejaculate volume and force can often be restored to more youthful levels.

Depending on the age and activity level, a man may experience shorter or longer refractory periods during the resolution stage of sex. As a result, some are ready for sexual activity again sooner than others.

The male orgasm appears to have psychological as well as physical effects. Research shows that men describe a focal experience, feeling the orgasm exclusively in the scrotum and genital area. Other men report feeling their orgasm as a sensation that spreads throughout their body.

During orgasm, as a man nears climax, his pelvic thrusts become less voluntary and the muscles in the penis begin to contract rhythmically in order to eject semen from the urethra. When the orgasm begins, a man's heart rate, blood pressure, and respiration all increase.

Once orgasm occurs, an increased infusion of the hormone oxytocin is released in the body. This hormone is thought to be responsible for the refractory period and the amount of the hormone that is released is believed to impact the length of each refractory period. Another chemical released during the refractory period is prolactin, which represses dopamine (a hormone that is responsible for the man's sexual arousal). This can also help explain the refractory period between male orgasms. Having prolactin levels checked as part of a comprehensive hormone evaluation is essential.

Research shows that a man's brain deactivates during his climax (but to a lesser extent than a women's) and brain scans have shown that the pleasure centers of a man's brain shows more intense activity during climax than a woman's.

The brain wave pattern shows distinct changes during sexual climax and a temporary decrease in metabolic activity or large parts of the cerebral cortex with increased metabolic activity in the limbic areas. Other research shows that the connection between orgasm and endorphins causes the body to produce natural "highs" that will help stabilize relations between couples.

The Physical Elements of the Male Orgasm

The male erection and orgasm is slightly more complicated than the penis. It involves various body parts working together to make the penis fully function.

There are several blood vessels in a man's pelvic area that supply blood to the lower half of the body, including some that just reach the male reproductive organs. The femoral artery and femoral vein travel through the pelvic bone to carry blood to and from a man's legs. Each of these has arteries and veins that branch out to supply blood to the penis. As you can see on Diagram D, the internal pudendal artery is the main vessel that supplies oxygenated blood to this organ.

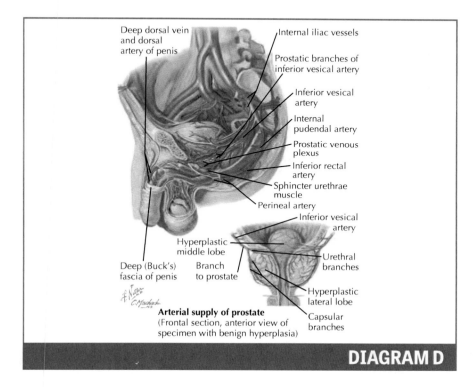

Deep dorsal vein and dorsal artery of penis

Internal iliac vessels

Prostatic branches of inferior vesical artery

Inferior vesical artery

Internal pudendal artery

Prostatic venous plexus

Inferior rectal artery

Sphincter urethrae muscle

Perineal artery

Inferior vesical artery

Hyperplastic middle lobe

Deep (Buck's) fascia of penis

Branch to prostate

Urethral branches

Hyperplastic lateral lobe

Capsular branches

Arterial supply of prostate
(Frontal section, anterior view of specimen with benign hyperplasia)

DIAGRAM D

Without proper function of this artery, a man could not achieve an erection. Problems with blood flow in this artery can cause erectile dysfunction.

In additional to arteries, there are several nerves that can impact a man's sexual function. Important nerves in the penile area include the pudendal nerve that reaches into external genitalia, the bladder, and rectum. The dorsal nerve of the penis is also important as it is the deepest branch of the pudendal nerve and responsible for the motor functions and sensation of the penis's skin.

The dorsal nerve of the penis is critical for erection. The brain sends a signal to the dorsal nerve of the penis to increase blood flow. This is also the nerve that receives the physical stimulation to achieve orgasm and ejaculation. If this nerve is damaged, a man's sexual experience can be seriously dampened.

It is important to understand that a male erection is achieved solely through pressurized blood. The penis can be limp or erect depending on how much blood flow it is receiving. An erection occurs when blood is trapped in the corpora cavernosa, causing the penis to elongate and stiffen. So, again, proper blood flow into the penis is pivotal for achieving erection.

What Can Go Wrong?

Sexual dysfunction in men is something that often impacts physical health, by bringing on depression, anxiety, and debilitating feelings of inadequacy. Furthermore, sexual problems can lead to relationship problems — either from lack of communications or understanding. The way a man feels about himself sexually is of paramount importance to his self-esteem. Men are expected to perform sexually well into old age. Every man with change in sexual function feels significant impact both psychologically and physically.

If sexual problems only occur under a particular set of circumstances or only with a particular sexual partner, the patient's condition is termed "situational" rather than "generalized." A man will experience many of these conditions on a temporary basis over the course of his life. Some healthcare professionals will only categorize the problem as sexual dysfunction if the condition persists twenty-five percent or more during all attempted sexual encounters. In the wider medical community, if a man's sexual problems are generalized and occurring at high frequency, this can be enough to diagnose him with a sexual disorder.

In my practice, a man or a woman does not "qualify" for the Priapus Shot™ or the O-Shot™. If there is a desire to improve the sexual experience or preserve the sexual experience, then the shot is warranted. While a man's orgasm might get more attention than a woman's, I believe it is just as important that he enjoy his entire sexual experience. Whether he has an issue obtaining an erection or simply orgasms more quickly than he would like (prior to his partner's satisfaction for instance), I want to help him achieve improved sexual wellness.

If you think you may be experiencing sexual dysfunction, take the following quiz:

Sexual Dysfunction Quiz for Men

- Do you experience difficulty in obtaining or maintaining an erection?
- Do you regularly reach climax before you or your partner is satisfied with your sexual experience?
- Do you often fail to reach climax?
- Can you only achieve orgasm after long periods of sexual stimulation?
- Have you experienced a decrease in erection firmness?

- Is your sexual desire significantly lower than it once was or even non-existent?

- Do you have a lack of ejaculation when you reach climax or lower ejaculate volume?

- Are you experiencing bloody ejaculations?

- Do you have painful or persistent erections unrelated to sexual desire?

- Do you have urinary issues such as:

    a. Frequent urination?

    b. Pain with urination?

    c. Night time urination?

    d. Difficulty stopping and/or starting a urinary stream?

If you answered yes to any of these questions, then you might be experiencing sexual dysfunction. In order to properly identify the root of the problem and offer proper treatment, it is important to understand the origin. Consider the following categories of sexual dysfunction:

Erectile Dysfunction (ED)

This condition is often referred to as impotence and is defined as the inability to have or maintain an erection sufficient for sexual function. This problem can result from blockages in blood flow, hardening of arteries, damage to arteries or nerves, leaky veins, low levels of testosterone, side effects from medications and mood challenges; anxiety, fear, depression.

Since you probably achieved your first erection as a pre-teen and have had multiple erections, several times a day since then — even at times when you did not want one or it was embarrassing to get caught with one — you have probably never thought of an erection as difficult to achieve. That is, until you started experiencing erectile dysfunction.

A series of mechanisms work together in order for a man to achieve a successful erection. When a man is aroused, nerves fire in his brain sending messages down the spinal cord to the penis. At that point, muscles relax and blood flows into the penis making it rigid. Anything that can interrupt this process — particularly the nerves and blood flow — can cause erectile dysfunction.

In later chapters the causes of all male sexual dysfunction is explained in greater detail, but in broad strokes, there are several contributing factors that can cause ED:

- Severe physical injuries
- Vascular diseases
- Smoking
- High blood pressure
- Diabetes
- High cholesterol
- Medications
- Poor Diet
- Hormone imbalance

Often erectile changes occur well before a man is diagnosed with cardiovascular disease, diabetes, etc. The symptom of erectile dysfunction should be taken seriously. While there are many simple and complex treatments to deal with erectile dysfunction, I recommend a blend of natural solution strategies that can preserve sexual function and even rehabilitate from significant dysfunction. This comprehensive approach is most successful when balance is re-established to the body. Harmful toxins should be removed and replaced with healthy habits, moderate exercise and a high density nutrient rich diet. In addition, I recommend PRP therapy as a means to improve the quality and potential of sexual response.

Ejaculation Problems

Ejaculatory disorders differ from erectile dysfunction. In these incidents a man can achieve an erection and engage in sex, but there is difficulty with the ejaculate. These disorders fall into three categories: premature ejaculation, inhibited ejaculation, and retrograde ejaculation.

Premature Ejaculation

Premature ejaculation can occur as a one-off incident for men of all ages, particularly if there has been long periods of time between sexual encounters or being over-excited by the situation or partner. Other factors that can cause the condition include past traumatic events, nervousness regarding performance, and certain medications. When the condition becomes chronic, the diagnosis is ejaculation that occurs before or soon after penetration.

It's important not to confuse what constitutes real "premature release" with perceived notions of "too soon". According to research, men typically reach orgasm between five and ten minutes after the start of penile-vaginal intercourse (Waldinger, MD 2005). Depending on the amount of time dedicated to foreplay, the time to orgasm might lengthen or shorten.

Do not make the mistake and believe you are experiencing "premature ejaculation" just because you cannot last an hour. (An hour would not be ***normal*** by any stretch of the imagination.)

That being said, it's important that you meet your own expectations. There are treatments available that will help maintain an erection for up to two to three hours safely, even after you ejaculate. The treatment strategy is called Intra-Cavernosal Pharmacology (ICP). ICP will be explained in detail in a later section.

Inhibited/Retarded Ejaculation

Inhibited or retarded ejaculation is essentially the opposite of premature ejaculation. It is diagnosed when the ejaculation is very slow to occur, takes a long time or simply does not occur at all. If a man can still ejaculate normally during masturbation, but not during intercourse, he can still be diagnosed with this condition.

This is one of those instances where a man might end up faking an orgasm. If it only happens once and awhile, it can probably be blamed on anxiety or other psychological factors. An isolated incident is not likely cause for concern; the cause might be an evening of overindulgence with alcohol. But if the problem persists, it can leave a man feeling very dissatisfied with sexual relations and might cause him to withdraw from intimacy with his partner. When the problem happens frequently, it is time to seek medical help.

The desire for a sexual marathon that exhausts your partner is not necessarily a good thing. Most couples simply do not have time for that much sexual interaction and a woman might start to feel like something is wrong with her if she cannot bring a man to climax. Mutual masturbation could prove helpful in the short-term, but couples will likely have a more meaningful sexual bond if they seek other treatments to solve the problem.

There are several potential causes when inhibited ejaculation becomes chronic (Laumann EO 1999):

- Physical damage
- Drug impairment
- Porn related issues
- Physiological issues
- Idiosyncratic condition
- Hormone Imbalance
- Aging tissue with decreased potential to respond to stimulus

It might seem odd or overly puritan to say that viewing porn could have a negative impact on a man's sexual performance, but research indicates it could be the case. The article, "Porn-Induced Sexual Dysfunction Is a Growing Problem" published in Psychology Today in 2011, Marnia Robinson details research and antidotal evidence of the problem (Robinson 2011). Research suggests that the overuse of porn can cause all sorts of issues, from overstimulation of the penis to misfires in dopamine in the brain.

There are of course, many other potential causes for this condition. Fear or psychological worries, neurological diseases, use of both prescription and recreational drugs, and conditions such as prostate infections can all lead to inhibited ejaculation. Consulting your doctor regarding your medications, decreasing alcohol consumption, and making some changes in your sexual habits can all help -as does open communication and honesty with both your partner and your doctor.

A decrease in penile sensitivity can be improved with the Priapus Shot™ (PRP) by regenerating the physiologic potential of the male sexual system.

Retrograde Ejaculation

Retrograde ejaculation is a condition with slightly more cause for concern than the first two mentioned in this section. It is sometimes referred to as a "dry orgasm." During climax, the ejaculation does not emerge from the penis, but is instead forced back into the bladder. This happens because of a failure of a normal bodily function. Normally, the sphincter of a man's bladder contracts before he orgasms and ejaculates, forcing his semen to exit through the urethra in his penis. If this sphincter fails to contract, seminal fluids enters the bladder instead.

Potential causes for this condition include damage to the nervous system and prostate. It can happen as a result of surgery, treatment for cancer, certain diseases, trauma to the pelvic area, or even certain types of medications. The most common types of medications that cause Retrograde Ejaculation are antidepressants and antipsychotic drugs (**www.mayoclinic.com**).

Treatments for this condition can include surgery or specific medications taken an hour or two prior to intercourse. For family planning, the couple might need to seek infertility treatments and in-vitro fertilization.

Priapism

Priapism is a condition related to ejaculation problems and is described best as a prolonged erection unaccompanied by sexual desire. If a man is unable to relieve the erection the condition can be potentially dangerous and requires immediate medical attention.

There are two classifications of priapism: low flow and high flow. Upwards of eighty percent of incidents are a result of low flow disorders, according to the *International Brazilian Journal of Urology* (Horst 2003). The low flow condition involves blood not properly returning to the body from the organ while the high flow condition occurs when there is a short-circuit of the vascular system pathway along the penis.

Causes for Priaprism can include diseases, medications, trauma to the spinal cord or genital areas, black widow spider bites, carbon monoxide poisoning, and the use of recreational drugs.

Treatment for Priapism can begin with ice packs to reduce swelling and pseudoephedrine to resolve the erection. If erection does not resolve with simple measures, invasive surgical procedures or shunts may be necessary. If the erection lasts more than four hours, then get to the Emergency Room immediately.

Painful Intercourse

Men can experience pain during intercourse for several reasons, including an infection of the prostate, urethra, or testes which can be independent or related to sexually transmitted diseases such as Chlamydia or genital herpes.

Some diseases, such as Peyronie's or fibrous plagues on the upper side of the penis, can often create a painful bend during erection. Other contributing factors can include an allergic reaction to condoms or spermicide as well as arthritis of the lower back.

Male Orgasmic Disorder

Male orgasmic disorder (MOD) can be defined as a recurrent inability to reach climax during intercourse or as a lack of ability to achieve orgasm without very lengthy sexual engagement. This condition can also be classified as the inability to reach climax during intercourse, but rather the man can only orgasm during masturbation or oral sex.

The man's inability to reach climax during a normal sexual cycle can be caused by several conditions, including both physical factors and psychological reasons. While diagnosing this condition, a doctor might perform a general physical examination, certain laboratory tests, and perhaps special tests to identify the underlying cause of the condition.

Potential causes of MOD include the following:

- Hypogonadism (the testes do not produce enough testosterone)
- Thyroid disorders
- Pituitary conditions
- Damage to the nervous system
- Substance abuse
- Some medications
- Depression
- Lack of emotional wellness
- High stress factors or fear
- Past sexual abuse

In additional to specific symptoms impacting sexual function, such as inability or delay in reaching orgasm, most patients with this condition complain of anxiety, guilt, shame, and bodily complaints. Part of diagnosing this condition is distinguishing this disorder from issues such as delayed or retrograde ejaculation.

The main difference is that in both of those conditions, orgasm occurs and in MOD, it usually does not.

Inhibited Sexual Desire/Low Libido

A decrease in sex drive can develop due to medical conditions and psychological or emotional factors; these include physical illness, hormonal abnormality (usually low testosterone levels), medications, or psychological causes.

Scientifically, low libido is categorized by a disinterest in sexual contact or complete lack of sexual desire. While a decrease in libido for a previously active man can be a result of any number of conditions, it is largely associated with low levels of testosterone.

Other factors that can inhibit a man's sexual desire include:

- Stress derived from work, financial problems, and other day-to-day worries
- Lack of sleep and/or deep fatigue
- Unresolved relationship issues Alcohol and recreational drugs
- Sleep Apnea
- Medications
- Obesity
- Depression

No matter the underlying cause, low libido can often be corrected by making healthy decisions and regaining some balance in life.

Relaxation techniques in dealing with stress and better sleep can prove beneficial, as can open communication with a spouse or partner. In addition, restorative medical treatments like bio-identical testosterone hormone replacement and Priapus Shot™ (PRP therapy) to truly regain previous levels of sexual interest and pleasure would be helpful.

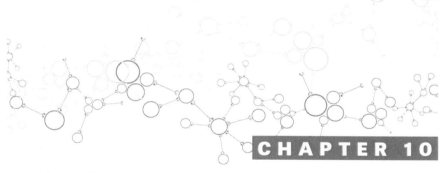

CHAPTER 10

Why & How to Seek Treatment

Sexual disorders carry varying stigmas and levels of embarrassment, therefore, many individuals never seek treatment. Even in my own practice as I treat men and women for symptoms of menopause and andropause, I am often the one who brings up the subject of sexual dysfunction.

Individuals often conclude that they can just "live with" these symptoms and it's a part of "growing old." Again, I want to assure all my readers that this simply is NOT true!

Reasons to Discuss Symptoms with Your Doctor

The most important reason for discussing your sexual health with your regular doctor is that sexual dysfunction is often a harbinger or symptom of a larger medical problem. If you are experiencing any of the signs or symptoms mentioned in this book, you should schedule an appointment with your physician.

Sexual dysfunction is not only a sign of potentially larger health issues, it can also impact other areas of your life. If you are having sexual problems with your significant other, feelings of unattractiveness can seep into your mindset and lead to depression. If you can identify sexual dysfunction as a source of negative feelings, you might be able to address the issue without the need for medications.

Another reason to talk to your regular doctor is that some sexual issues might be caused by medications for conditions such as high blood pressure. By discussing the fact that you are experiencing sexual dysfunctions, your doctor may be able to identify an alternative dose or prescription that will not interfere with your sexual activities.

Once you create an open dialogue, it will be easier to figure out if an expert is needed in areas of hormone therapy or PRP treatments.

Why You Should Consult an Expert

As previously mentioned, the treatment course I prefer to take for sexual dysfunction is more expansive than many of my colleagues. Essentially, it encompasses all sexual dissatisfaction. It is not necessary for a woman to have a pre-existing condition that prevents her from having sex to seek treatment; she just needs to be dissatisfied with the quality of her sexual experience.

Additionally, a man only needs to be dissatisfied with any part of his sexual performance.

Using PRP to improve and preserve sexual function is a very exciting protocol and has satisfied my patients with reaching their sexual performance goals. I continue to be amazed with the overwhelming positive results.

If your doctor does not consider your condition serious enough for treatment, working with an expert might prove beneficial. Another reason to work with a specialist is for hormone therapy. I realize that many general practitioners will prescribe hormone treatments, particularly testosterone for men. However, how much and how effectively they prescribe these medicines is questionable. If you find that your testosterone or estrogen levels are off, you should work with a specialist who understands how both hormones work together and how you can achieve an optimal balance that will benefit you sexually, as well as for your general health.

The Importance of Treatment for Individuals

Aside from your physical health, sexual dysfunction can negatively impact many other aspects of your life, from relationships to self-confidence to stress levels. The truth is, all forms and all severity of sexual dysfunction can have damaging effects on your physical and emotional health, as well as your quality of life.

When it comes to sex, if a man or woman is experiencing discomfort or difficulty, he or she might become less likely to try to engage in the activity itself. Lack of activity or anxiety over poor performance can make the underlying issue even worse. As a result, sexual dysfunction can transform from physical or pharmaceutical problem to one that includes psychological obstacles.

While open communications with your partner can help to lessen a troubling self-esteem, not everyone is comfortable being this open. At the very least, addressing your sexual problems with your doctor should facilitate treatment.

Stress Relief

Sexual activity is often associated with the release of hormones that have positive effects on both men and women. As a result, reaching climax during sexual engagement acts as a stress release for both genders.

While this is certainly a positive impact of sexual functions, the absence of or difficulty in achieving climax can prove highly stressful on both men and women. As described above, sexual dysfunction can place undue burden or pressure on a relationship, which affects the individual and amplifies the original condition. In a nutshell, sexual problems make sexual problems worse.

Successful treatment for sexual dysfunction lowers the stress levels for individuals as well as relationships.

Quality of Life

Over the last 15 years, it has become more and more acceptable that middle-aged couples have active sex lives beyond their child-bearing years. While this seems like a revolutionary concept, to myself and my colleagues, people of all ages *should* be able to enjoy a healthy sex life.

Of course, with the "free-love" generation reaching AARP-membership age, there is little wonder oral medications prescribed to treat erectile dysfunction became a multibillion-dollar industry. Yet there is so much more to sexual health than treatments for ED. It's necessary that both men — and women — seek sexual wellness in order to fully enjoy a high quality of life.

I should also note, since sexual hindrances are so closely aligned with female incontinence, seeking treatment such as the O-Shot™ can improve the quality of life in unimaginable ways. The link between depression and incontinence is well established in women; solving this problem invites a phenomenal outlook on life.

The Importance of Treatment for Couples

While there are many reasons for individuals to seek treatment, I think there is tremendous benefit for couples who seek treatment together, if one or both experience difficulties. I see this often in my practice; one patient comes to me for help and more often, I end up treating the partner as well. The O-Shot™ and Priapus

Shot™ for couples brings them closer together and strengthens their bond.

A healthy sexual relationship is an important part of intimacy, at any age. It's very important for those experiencing the "empty nest" to maintain a thriving intimate relationship. Too many marriages fail because couples physically grow apart.

Hormones released in the brain upon climax triggers the desire to attach or "cuddle." This one fact can keep intimacy growing strong over a life-long relationship. Sex is possible without intimacy and vice versa, but the chemical reaction when sharing a sexual experience plays an important role.

A Note for Women

In 1989, the character Sally, from "When Harry Met Sally" let the cat out of the bag when she faked an orgasm in a New York restaurant. Research indicates that up to eighty percent of women admit to faking orgasms with their partners (Alexander 2010).

The reasons women fake orgasms range from being stressed to feeling over weight. It's a wonder to know if some women truly have sexual dysfunction.

When a problem with sexual function persists beyond a temporary condition caused by stress or other life conditions, a chronic condition can have a negative impact on a woman's self-confidence, her relationship with her partner, and her overall health.

Remember that the list of "causes" of sexual changes can be quite extensive. Sometimes sexual changes can be the first and only sign of an underlying problem. Often if these "problems" are not addressed they can worsen and cause serious health changes.

As discussed in the previous section, a women's orgasm releases several positive hormones into her system. It is also considered a large source of tension release and relaxation. Can women live without these health benefits? Certainly. But the relationship bond will suffer and the possibility of additional problems will increase. It's very important that women take the proactive approach and open the dialog with a health professional.

A healthy sexual desire and function are part of a healthy body, mind and spirit. Sexual energy is a powerful force that women can learn to harness in order to bring joy, stability, strength and balance to their lives and beyond. Sexual intimacy between partners is a powerful connection that keeps families together; and what is shared in private often over flows into the world, at large.

Regarding Incontinence

Incontinence can lead to a complete lack of desire for sexual activity — or any other physical activity. Fear of embarrassment is a natural hindrance to self-confidence and it can lead to avoiding social settings and exercise. The potential for low self-esteem and depression increases as does the incontinence.

Proper treatment allows a woman greater sexual freedom, improved social interaction, and independence. Eliminating the ever-persistent worry about going out in public is so important.

We easily recognize that stress and/or urge incontinence can negatively affect the quality of life. More people accept this condition as something aging individuals (women in particular) have to accept — and it's simply not true. Furthermore, since the correlation between depression and incontinence go hand in hand, it is important to be proactive and seek treatment.

The No. 1 reason a woman is admitted to the nursing home is urinary incontinence.

It's very interesting, the family will find ways to take care of her when she is physically and mentally failing, but once she becomes incontinent, a whole host of care giving challenges arise. Sadly, she is better cared for in a nursing home.

Urinary incontinence is not only a progressive disease, but also devastating in regards to elderly care. The FACT is -urinary incontinence is treatable and deserves more respect and attention. The longer urinary incontinence goes untreated, the more difficult it is to resolve.

I have helped many women overcome the most challenging cases of incontinence with using the regenerative power of PRP and effective, in home, pelvic bowl rehabilitation.

A Note for Men

The positive effects of sexual well-being are profoundly documented. Yet, discussing sexual problems with a doctor can be embarrassing and a difficult conversation to start. Admitting to sexual problems equates to a lack of manhood. And men often feel that they are alone in their experience.

Many feel sexual dysfunction is a sign aging and 'too old' to perform. I've heard several men joke, "You know it's over when you have to take the little blue pill." The truth is, many men experience sexual problems at an age when they still want to be sexually active (40's and 50's). Up to 31 percent of ALL men report sexual problems such as erectile dysfunction and premature ejaculation.

For more than two decades, the idea of women faking orgasms has been known. However, in 2010 men were also reported to faking orgasms (Muehlenhard 2010). According to Muehlenhard's study, twenty-five percent of men and fifty percent of women fake away.

Why men? Despite the ability for a man to experience a dry orgasm, we tend to associate a man's climax with ejaculation. So how can that be faked?

Not all sexual dysfunction results in the inability to get erect. Sometimes, it can be manifested in an inability to reach climax or very low ejaculation. Other times, an erection may occur, but not be sustained. With the use of a condom, it can be easy to fake a climax without the woman becoming suspicious. Even without using a condom, a woman might not notice a slight ejaculation (or absence of ejaculation).

Men report the need to fake an orgasm for much of the same reasons women do; an inability to climax, a desire not to disappoint his/her partner, a desire to end the sexual act early, and a fear of embarrassment.

The problem — or one of the problems — with faking an orgasm for both sexes is that it means one person is hiding something significant. While a man may not want to admit this to his partner, it will ultimately cause of lack of intimacy and eventual emotional and physical withdrawal.

Therefore, even if a man is not prepared to discuss his sexual problems with his partner, he should at least discuss them with his doctor. Finding the appropriate treatment might require blood tests and a discussion of existing medical conditions and medicines. But with a proper exploration of health factors, finding a solution for sexual dysfunction is very possible. In fact, restoring sexual wellness for a man can be as simple as adjusting medicines or hormonal treatments. Both can bring many positive benefits to his life; energy, mood, motivation, strength, sleep, body composition, and self-esteem.

Because Treatments Work!

The most exciting reason I can give you to seek treatment for sexual dysfunction is because treatment works! Your sex life CAN improve. You CAN experience more desire, more intense arousal, better erections, heightened orgasms and more intimacy with sexual success and satisfaction.

In my practice, I design customized solutions for my clients to achieve their optimal health and sexual well-being. These solutions can involve many factors: bio-identical hormone replacement therapy, diet changes, exercise and regenerative strategies. Additionally, I use platelet-rich plasma treatments to encourage tissue healing and rejuvenation. This exciting new treatment is full of potential.

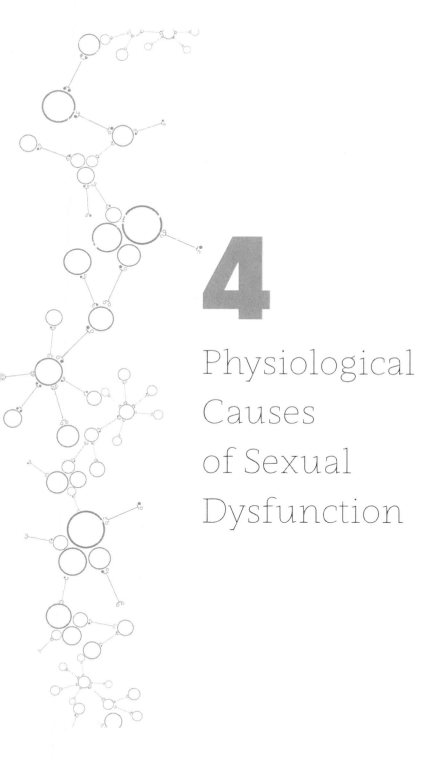

4

Physiological Causes of Sexual Dysfunction

While many people think of sexual dysfunction as a natural sign of aging, the truth is that sexual dysfunction can act precisely like the proverbial "canary in the cave." Sexual problems in men and women are almost always a symptom of another condition of some sort. These conditions can include hormonal changes in a man or woman's body, disease, medication, or any number of traumatic events that damage tissue or muscles in the pelvic area.

As you know by now, I define sexual dysfunction as "any change in sexual function that leaves the individual or their partner with a less than satisfactory sexual experience." This means that you could experience any number of the causal issues described in this part of the book and still be perfectly satisfied with your sex life.

With that said, the causes of sexual dysfunction are vast and common and explained in Part Three. Hopefully, readers will be encouraged to take action.

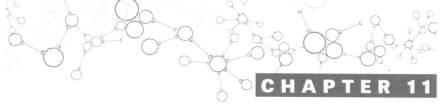

CHAPTER 11

Hormonal Changes as a Cause of Sexual Dysfunction

As men and women age, they will both experience hormonal changes that can negatively impact sexual dysfunction. When women go through menopause or have a complete hysterectomy, a decrease in estrogen naturally occurs. Many men also experience a decrease in hormone (testosterone) levels as they enter their "middle aged" years.

When examining the issues of hormonal changes, it is important to understand what changed and why. Once identified, a physician should be able to provide an ideal strategy for optimizing levels to increase energy and sexual activity.

Thyroid Imbalance

The thyroid gland produces and regulates hormones that affect energy levels, growth and development, mood (depression), sexual functions, reproduction, and metabolism (weight). When the thyroid does not produce enough hormones, the body uses energy at a slower pace which can cause any of the following:

- Dry, coarse skin and hair
- Fatigue
- Forgetfulness
- Frequent or heavy menstrual flows
- Hoarse voice
- Sensitivity to cold
- Weight gain
- Enlargement of the thyroid gland

Until recently, the connection between sexual dysfunction and thyroid disease was suspected but not proven. However, as early as 2005, a study published in the Journal of Clinical Endocrinology and Metabolism, researchers established a connection between specific sexual problems in men and thyroid conditions, including hypothyroidism and hyperthyroidism (Shomon 2013).

The study looked at 48 adult men who were evaluated for a number of common problems, including low sex drive, erectile dysfunction, premature ejaculation, and delayed ejaculation. They were examined while symptomatic, and again once their thyroid levels returned to a normal range.

The study concurred that more than sixty-four percent of symptomatic patients of hypothyroid men complained of erectile dysfunction. In addition, fifty percent experienced premature ejaculation, seventeen percent complained of low sex drive, and fourteen percent reported erectile dysfunction.

Once treatment began and the thyroid function returned to normal, most sexual symptoms completely reversed.

Thyroid disease and sexual concerns for women are not as easily addressed. Reports show that women still complained of low sex drive even after their thyroid returned to normal levels. Some medical experts believe those particular cases arose prior to seeking thyroid treatment.

As many as ten percent of women over the age of 50 have some degree of thyroid hormone deficiency, with low thyroid production being the most common issue (**www.webmd.com**). Along with fatigue, muscle aches, and depression, decreased sexual desire is also considered a symptom of the disease.

Advice for women with thyroid conditions includes, balancing estrogen and progesterone hormones, optimal testosterone levels, weight loss, nutritional supplements, and exercise. Weight loss and exercise in particular can prove to be helpful. Research shows that a mere 10 to 20 pound weight loss reduces enough body fat to lower the levels of sex hormone binding globulin (SHBG) that blocks estrogen production (**www.webmd.com**). Since the fatigue can lead to weight gain, once treatment has proven successful, exercise can help take off the extra pounds and improve hormone production.

Low Testosterone

It is common knowledge that a woman's hormones change as she goes through menopause, but men at large are unaware that testosterone levels decrease as a natural function of aging. Physicians at Mayo Clinic conducted studies showing after the age of 30, testosterone levels decrease at a rate of one percent per year. (**www.mayoclinic.com**).

It is important to state that testosterone is the most abundant biologically active hormone in women as well as men. Testosterone plays a vital role in normal development, and optimal wellness; physically, mentally, sexually, and metabolically. Many aspects of optimal living are affected by declining testosterone levels in both men and women.

A decrease in sex drive is often the first sign of low testosterone. Of course, between career pursuits, changes in sexual activity (perhaps due to parenthood), and other factors can decrease sexual desires in couples between their 30's and 40's. Many men may not even notice this initial decline.

However, there are other side-effects of low testosterone that men might begin to notice cumulatively. Signs include changes in sperm production, muscle mass and strength, fat distribution, bone density, and red blood cell production.

Sexual dysfunction associated with low testosterone include low libido and erectile dysfunction. Additionally, some men experience infertility. Other physical changes that can negatively impact a man's sexual interest are listed below.

Increase in Body Fat

As a man ages and his physical activity decreases, weight gain is fairly normal. However, for a man who maintains the same amount of physical activity yet his weight becomes an issue, low testosterone could be the culprit.

Decrease in Muscle Mass

If a man is in the practice of lighting weights or working out, he might find that it becomes increasingly difficult to maintain muscular definition. If a man is less likely to work out, he might become unusually flabby. Testosterone is key to building and maintaining muscles. This change might not be a product of one too many donuts; it could be a sign of a change in the body's chemical makeup.

Fragile Bones

Hopefully, a broken or fractured bone is not the tip off you get to have your testosterone levels checked. Hormones are is vital in building a man's bone density. The development of fragile or weak bones is common with low testosterone.

Loss of Hair

The connection between low testosterone and hair loss is more complex than some of the other symptoms discussed, but it's something to consider. Male pattern baldness affects seventy percent of men in their lives (Case-Lo 2013). But testosterone imbalance does not just impact the hair on the head; it can also create changes in facial and chest hair.

Tender/Enlarged Breast Tissue

As men gain weight and either lose muscle mass or never develop it, they are often jokingly referred to as having "man boobs." However, gynecomastia is a real medical condition producing tender and enlarged breast tissue in men. The condition presents itself as rubbery or formed mass starting under the nipple and then spreading over the breast area (**www.andrologyaustralia. org**).

In reality, gynecomastia is not a result of fat tissue, but enlargement of glandular tissue. Men of any age can experience the condition and the tissue that grows is often tender or painful to the touch. When younger men experience this condition, it often goes away over time. But in older men, about thirty-three percent experience a chronic condition (**www.andrologyaustralia.org**). Balancing testosterone levels should help elevate this condition.

Increased Fatigue

Some men experience decreased energy with low testosterone. Others can experience sleep disturbances including insomnia. In either situation, increased fatigue throughout a normal day warrants testing.

Hot Flashes

You might think I have mixed up my sections with this last symptom, but it's true — men can experience discomfort from flushing and sweating caused by hot flashes. If you are going through andropause, the male menopause, this might be one of the most significant warning signs. According to a study conducted at Harvard, up to eighty percent of men treated for androgen deprivation therapy experience this symptom (**www.health.harvard. edu**).

While some antidepressant medications have been known to relieve hot flashes, hormonal therapies have been twice as effective and come with benefits for sexual function rather than potential obstacles (Irani 2010).

Emotional Changes

A man with significantly decreased testosterone can also experience emotional changes, including depression, low motivation, low self-confidence and even issues with memory or concentration.

All of these factors could have a negative effect on a man's sex drive and a loss of libido could create any of these feelings. As a result, low testosterone is important to discuss with a doctor for general wellness and quality of life.

Thanks to the launch of Viagra in 1998, and all related medications that followed, the stigma regarding male sexual problems has largely diminished. However, men still might feel uncomfortable speaking to their doctor about "hormones" — something that is largely thought of as a "female issue."

Yet medical researchers looking to duplicate the wild success of Viagra have pushed on in pursuit for the "next big thing" and developed several low testosterone treatments. Companies are advertising Low-T treatments on a mass scale.

Low-T advertisements layout the symptoms of low testosterone quite well and tell men exactly what to talk about to their doctors. An easy blood test can confirm what the patient suspects and then it is just a matter of determining which treatment delivery is best for the individual; Testosterone Pellet Therapy, creams, or injectable products. Since odds are good that any man over the age of 30 will be experiencing Low-T to one degree or another, the advertisers of these products have good odds of making the sale.

Treatments for low testosterone can include monthly shots, daily gels, or pellets which are implanted under the skin and release hormones gradually over the course of several months. There are some medical conditions — such as breast and prostate cancer — that might prohibit testosterone replacement therapy so a complete physical examination might be advisable before beginning treatment.

Low Estrogen/Progesterone

Estrogen and progesterone are the female sex hormones. Estrogen acts as the catalyst to transition a girl's body into a more-womanly figure. It also stimulates the sympathetic nervous system, increases alertness, lowers body fat, and protects against heart and Alzheimer's disease. Estrogen is also known to improve insulin sensitivity and improve glucose tolerance.

During reproductive years, a woman makes estrogen every day of the month. The ovaries also produce progesterone during the two weeks before a woman's period. Progesterone reduces anxiety, has a calming effect on mood, and essentially makes a woman happy. It also improves sleep, helps build and maintain bones, slows the digestive process, promotes appetite, helps breast tissue mature, and prepares breasts to produce milk at the end of a pregnancy.

Menopause has an influence on hormone levels, causing one or both to fall. However, a decrease in one hormone can occur at other times during the reproductive years. When this happens, a woman is likely to experience some form of sexual dysfunction. The first step in recognizing low hormone levels in a woman is an examination of common symptoms and include:

Irregular or Absent Menstruation

While the sign for menopause in women is a change in their menstrual cycle, younger women who experience this change should consult a specialist immediately as it can signal a larger problem.

Mood Changes/Problems

Estrogen and progesterone both affect mood and therefore low levels of either hormone can cause irritability and depression. Low estrogen tends to result in sadness or depressed feelings while low progesterone is more likely to result in an agitated, worried state of mind with a tendency toward mood swings.

When either of these hormones dips lower than it should, a woman can also experience trouble sleeping and suffer from feelings of fatigue.

Weight Gain

Hormone levels have an influence with weight gain and water retention. Women with low levels of estrogen might experience a decrease in breast size while women with low progesterone might find their breasts have enlarged. Women might also experience bloating or tender/sore breasts.

Weight gain around the hips and abdomen is also common for women with low levels of estrogen or progesterone. Too little estrogen can result in an overall weight gain and fat accumulation around the stomach, changing a woman's body into an "apple" shape.

Sexual Dysfunction

Besides the fact that the above conditions can impact a woman's desire to have sex, low levels of estrogen and progesterone can also decrease the libido and vaginal lubrication. When these hormone decrease, a woman is also more likely to contract vaginal infections which can damper her ability to engage in sexual activity.

Outside of menopause, there are several other reasons why women of all ages could experience low levels of estrogen and/or progesterone, including the following:

Surgical Events

Many women experience changes in sexual function after a partial or full hysterectomy (the surgical removal of the uterus). Those changes can include loss of desire, decreased vaginal lubrication, and genital sensation. The removal of the uterus can impact hormonal levels and the nerves/blood vessels critical to sexual function.

Low Natural Production

There are three types of estrogen: estriol, estradiol, and estrone. Some women do not naturally produce enough of one or all forms of the hormone. Abnormal levels of one or more could signal the presence of ovarian or adrenal cancer or conditions such as cysts on or in the ovaries.

Pregnancy Related Conditions

Pregnancy, childbirth, and breast-feeding is a sequence of events that severely impact a woman's body and hormone levels. In some cases, a significant decrease in estrogen in young women can signal pregnancy problems that could lead to a miscarriage. The condition can also be present during/after childbirth and breast-feeding.

Eating Disorders and/or Excessive Exercise

For a body to function properly and produce the appropriate levels of hormones, there's a level of body fat that must be maintained. Significantly less body fat interrupts the menstrual cycle and influences the appearance of looking less "feminine."

Unhealthy Lifestyle Choices

Some women are candidates for hormone replacement therapy while others are not. However, there are lifestyle changes that can positively impact estrogen levels. These include maintaining a healthy diet with the addition of herbs, improving exercise, no tobacco, and limiting the use of caffeine to two cups of coffee a day.

CHAPTER 12

Sexual Changes Should be Considered "The Canary in the Cave." They are Often the First Symptom of a Serious Disease.

If you think of sexual dysfunction as being a symptom rather than a condition in and of itself, then you can see how it might connect to several diseases. Most likely if you have been diagnosed with diabetes or a heart condition, you already know that the disease (or the treatment for it) might negatively impact your sex life.

However, if you are experiencing sexual problems and do not know why, consider the conditions listed in this chapter. If you have any reason to be suspicious (even with family history) you should discuss the possibility with your doctor.

186 *Regenerating Sexual Potential*

Diabetes

Diabetes is a disease that affects the blood vessels (which can impede blood flow to the penis or vagina) and cause possible harm the nerves in the pelvic region. In men, diabetes can lead to hardening and narrowing of blood vessels that supply the erectile tissue of the penis. This can create problems with obtaining or maintaining erections.

In women, diabetes can lead to hardening or narrowing of blood vessels in the vaginal wall. Decreased blood flow can negatively impact vaginal lubrication — making sex uncomfortable or even painful. If women have sex in this situation, reports show they are at greater risk for recurring yeast infections.

For people with diabetes, the first step in treating sexual dysfunction is to control their blood glucose levels with a wellness focused whole food diet and targeted supplement strategy. When the condition is maintained, both men and women experience a decrease in complications, including sexual dysfunction. Additional treatment options range from PRP Treatment, oral medication to mechanical devices and lubricants.

Cardiovascular Conditions

Many cardiovascular diseases, especially hypertension and peripheral vascular disease, create changes in the small blood vessels that supply areas of the body such as legs, feet, and genitals. Poor blood flow to the penis or vagina can affect a person's ability to become aroused and engage in sexual intercourse. Research shows a large percentage of erectile dysfunction cases are the result of blood vessel related diseases.

Symptoms such as fatigue, shortness of breath, chest pain, and muscle weakness can be signs of cardiovascular disease and the symptoms alone can lower sex drive. In particular, the fear that sexual activity can trigger a cardio event can be a mental block to sexual function as well as a physical one.

Finally, medications that are prescribed to treat cardiovascular disease — particularly hypertension — are often associated with negative sexual side effects. These side effects can range from a loss of desire to erectile dysfunction and problems with ejaculation.

If you have been diagnosed with this condition, lifestyle changes to quit smoking, reduce alcohol intake, eat a healthy diet, and engage in regular exercise can help improve blood flow and reduce the occurrence of sexual problems. If additional treatments are necessary, discussing strategies and recommendations with your doctor.

High Blood Pressure

The link between high blood pressure and sexual dysfunction has been proven in men. Over time, high blood pressure damages the lining of blood vessels and causes arteries to harden and narrow, thereby limiting blood flow to the sex organs. For some men, the decreased blood flow makes it difficult to achieve and maintain erections, often referred to as erectile dysfunction.

Medications for high blood pressure can cause sexual dysfunction. Water pills (diuretics) can decrease blood flow to the penis, making it difficult for men to achieve an erection. These pills can also decrease the body's supply of zinc, which is necessary for testosterone production. Beta blockers are medications that can impact the nervous system reaction and the ability to achieve an erection.

Women with high blood pressure can lack sexual interest, but the connection is not well understood. However, high blood pressure can reduce blood flow to the vagina, thereby decreasing sexual desire, arousal, vaginal dryness, and the ability to experience orgasms.

Changes in medication, PRP Treatments, and other treatments can help compensate for patients with high blood pressure to restore normal sexual activity.

Lipid Disorders

Male patients with lipid disorders or high cholesterol/triglycerides report experiencing increased risk of erectile dysfunction. The treatment for this condition — often fibrates and statins — are also known to produced erective disorders.

High levels of cholesterol can also cause Coronary Artery Disease (CAD) which can further complicate sexual wellness, as can related conditions such as obesity and hypertension.

Atherosclerosis and Coronary Artery Disease

Hardening of the arteries (atherosclerosis) and Coronary Artery Disease (CAD) are both known to contribute to erectile dysfunction. The link between atherosclerosis and erectile dysfunction is well proven to doctors; understanding the connection can contribute to overall health and well-being.

In men, the blood supply to the penis comes from arteries in the abdomen. Smaller arteries branch off to carry blood down to the penis. As men become aroused, the arteries dilate and blood flows into the penis causing it to swell.

The rush of blood creates high pressure in the penis that also slows down the flow of blood out of the penis. If the blood vessels are healthy, this produces a firm erection that can be maintained until orgasm. When erectile dysfunction occurs, it means the blood vessels are not in perfect health – having either been hardened or weakened.

The inside lining of blood vessels (endothelium) releases chemicals on demand to create wide-open blood flow to the arteries in the heart. This section can be damaged by high cholesterol, high blood pressure, smoking, or diabetes. Once damaged, the endothelium cannot expand arteries to increase blood flow; less blood flow into the penis means a less firm erection.

Prostate Cancer

While any cancer patient undergoing chemotherapy and radiation treatments might experience a decrease in sexual interest, medicines used to treat prostate cancer in particular can cause ED.

First, surgical options can damage the nerves that effect and control erections. This is no reason to forgo surgery, but it is important to understand potential sources of concerns.

Second, radiation or hormone therapy can impact erectile function and libido levels. If a man desires to have sex during the period where he is receiving cancer treatment, there is a wide-range of options to help him overcome his sexual difficulties. Many of those will be examined in detail later in this book.

Parkinson's Disease

Sexual dysfunction is common among patients with Parkinson's disease. It is considered part of the deterioration process and their quality of life. Both men and women with this condition often report loss of desire.

Men and women can experience tremors, hypomania, muscle rigidity, bradykinesia, clumsiness in fine motor control, dyskinesia, hyper salivation, and sweating that can interfere with sexual activity. Hypo sexuality, erectile dysfunction, and problems with ejaculation occur in male patients; loss of lubrication and involuntary urination (incontinence) during sex are common for female patients.

Multiple Sclerosis

Individuals with Multiple Sclerosis (MS) often experience sexual difficulties because sexual arousal begins in the central nervous system. The brain sends messages to the sexual organs along nerves running through the spinal cord. If MS damages these nerve pathways, sexual response, arousal, and orgasm, is affected. Other MS symptoms, such as fatigue or spasticity as well as mood changes or depression, can negatively impact sexual functions.

Research has shown that as many as 63 percent of people with MS report that their sexual activity has decreased since their diagnosis. As many as ninety-one percent of men and seventy-two percent of women with MS admit to experiencing sexual problems (**www. nationalmssociety.org**).

In women, symptoms include reduced sensation in the vaginal/ clitoral area or painfully heightened sensation, as well as vaginal dryness, trouble achieving climax, and loss of libido. In men, symptoms include difficulty in achieving or maintaining erections, reduced penile sensation, difficulty in achieving orgasm and or ejaculation, and loss of libido.

General symptoms of MS can cause problems in men and women, including fatigue and weakness, spasticity (cramping or uncontrolled spasms in the legs), general pain, or bowel/bladder incontinence.

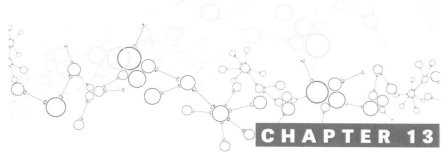

CHAPTER 13

Many Medications Can Cause Noticeable Changes in Sexual Function

If you are having problems achieving or maintaining an erection or experiencing any other sexual dysfunction described in earlier chapters of this book, one of the first items to discuss with your doctor are the medications you are taking for other conditions.

There are a number of prescriptions and over-the-counter drugs that can cause sexual complications. They can impact hormone levels (testosterone and estrogen), alter levels of chemicals in the brain, impact nerve functions and/or blood circulation, among other factors.

In this chapter, there is a comprehensive list of drug categories with generic and brand names (taken from WebMD) that you might want to discuss with your doctor. The possible side effects of these medications include decreased libidos (or sex drive), impotence or erectile dysfunction, delayed or absent orgasm, and ejaculatory disturbances (including low volume or delayed/failure to ejaculate).

Diuretics & High Blood Pressure Medications

An estimated seventy percent of men who experience side effects from taking high blood pressure medication -stop taking it- primarily because one of the most significant complications is erectile dysfunction. While this is understandable, it is still important to discuss this decision with your doctor. Certain drugs used to treat high blood pressure are less likely to cause this condition and some have been documented to improve erectile dysfunction (**www.webmd.com**).

The correlation between diuretics and beta-blockers and ED is well documented. However, if you are on one of these medications, you should first attempt to lower your blood pressure through diet and exercise before going off the medication altogether.

The list of diuretics and high blood pressure medicines that can cause sexual dysfunction include the following (generic and brand names):

- Hydrochlorothiazide (Esidrix, HydroDIURIL, Hydropres, Inderide, Moduretic, Oretic, Lotensin)
- Chlorthalidone (Hygroton)
- Triamterene (Maxide, Dyazide)
- Furosemide (Lasix)
- Bumetanide (Bumex)

- Guanfacine (Tenex)
- Methyldopa (Aldomet)
- Clonidine (Catapres)
- Verapamil (Calan, Isoptin, Verelan)
- Nifedipine (Adalat, Procardia)
- Hydralazine (Apresoline)
- Captopril (Capoten)
- Enalapril (Vasotec)
- Metoprolol (Lopressor)
- Propranolol (Inderal)
- Labetalol (Normodyne)
- Atenolol (Tenormin)
- Phenoxybenzamine (Dibenzyline)
- Spironolactone (Aldactone)

Some families of high blood pressure meds are less likely to cause erectile dysfunction and discussing those with your doctor as an alternative medicine might be the best place to start. These families include ACE inhibitors, Alpha-Blockers, Calcium Channel Blockers, and ARBs.

If you think your medication is causing your sexual difficulties, remember to keep taking the prescription until you can talk to your doctor about an alternative medicine. Also, remember that dietary changes and exercise can also lesson your need for high blood pressure medication.

Antidepressants, Anti-Anxiety, and Antiepileptic Medications

Sexual side effects are common with women and men who take antidepressants or anti-anxiety meds. The severity of the issue can depend on the individual and the dose of the medication prescribed. Some categories of drugs are more likely to cause problems than others. Therefore, if you are experiencing difficulties, it is important to discuss alternative solutions with your doctor or the possibility of taking a lower dose.

Antidepressants that are most likely to cause sexual side effects include:

- SSRIs (Selective Serotonin Reuptake Inhibitors)
- Citalopram (Celexa)
- Escitalopram (Lexapro)
- Fluoxetine (Prozac/Sarafem)
- Fluvoxamine (Luvox)
- Paroxetine (Paxil/Pexeva)
- Sertraline (Zoloft)
- SNRIs (Serotonin and Norepinephrine Reuptake Inhibitors)
- Venlafaxine (Effexor)
- Desvenlafaxine (Pristiq)
- Duloxetine (Cymbalta)
- Tricyclic & Tetracyclic Antidepressants
- Amitriptyline

- Clomipramine (Anafranil)
- Amoxapine
- Despiramine (Norpramin)
- Amoxipine (Asendin)
- MAOIs (Monoamine Oxidase Inhibitors)
- Tranylcypromine (Parnate)
- Isocarboxazid (Marplan)
- Phenelzine (Nardil)

The antidepressants with the lowest rate of sexual side effects include Burpropion (Wellbutrin), Amitriptyline (Elavil), and Mirtazapine (Remeron). If you are experiencing difficulties with any of the above medication, talk to your doctor about switching to one of these options.

Several of the medications used to treat depression are also prescribed to treat anxiety. If you have been prescribed one of the antidepressants listed above and want to switch to something else for your anxiety issues, talk to your doctor about one these medications: Bupropion, Mirtazapine, and Buspirone.

Antiepileptic drugs have long been associated with sexual disorders, but the causality is not certain. Sexual problems associated with epilepsy can occur with or without the onset of seizures. Common sexual disorders reported include hypo sexuality (lack of sexual desire) and the alteration of sex hormone levels. Discuss options with your doctor is you are on antiepileptic medication, but do not stop taking the prescribed drug as it could be a life-threatening choice.

Cholesterol Medications

By limiting the availability of cholesterol (a building block of hormones) in the body, drugs used to lower cholesterol can interfere with the production of testosterone, estrogen, and other sex hormones. Some statins can cause a breakdown of muscle tissue and fatigue, which can also inhibit sexual activity.

Studies have shown that both fibrates and statins can cause impotence and that men and women taking these medications report an increase of difficulty in achieving orgasms. However, not all statins are associated with sexual dysfunction and event those that are, the risk of developing the condition is low.

Therefore, if you are taking cholesterol medicine and encountering sexual difficulties, you can talk to your doctor about switching medications or using vitamins such as B12, Folic Acid, and B6. Fish oil has also been found to be instrumental in lowering cholesterol naturally. There are many dietary changes that focus on optimizing body composition that will have a positive effect. This discussion is beyond the scope of this book. Just know that cholesterol is not the enemy that we are led to believe.

Examples of cholesterol medications with reported sexual side effects include:

- Gemfibrozil (Lopid)

- Clofibrate
- Fenofibrate (TriCor/Lofibra)
- Simvastatin (Zocor)
- Atorvastatin (Lipitor)
- Rosuvastatin (Crestor)
- Lovastatin (Altoprev/Mevacor)
- Fluvastatin (Lescol)
- Pravastatin (Pravachol)

Antihistamines/Histamine H2-Receptor Antagonists

You might be surprised to learn that some common allergy medications with antihistamines (even the over-the-counter) can cause a temporary form of erectile dysfunction. If you are taking any of these medications and find yourself having difficulty maintaining an erection, try switching to an alternative over-the-counter medicine or talk to your doctor about a different prescription. It is important that you understand what is causing the histamine response:

- Dimehydrinate (Dramamine)
- Diphenhydramine (Benadryl)
- Hydroxyzine (Vistaril)
- Meclizine (Antivert)
- Promethazine (Phenergan)

Some antacids that are antihistamines, used to treat indigestion, acid reflux and GERD (Gastroesophagelal Reflux Disorder) have also been associated with temporary erectile dysfunction. Examples include:

- Cimetidine (Tagamet)
- Nizatidine (Axid)
- Ranitidine (Zantac)

Non-Steroidal Anti-Inflammatory Drugs

Research suggests there is a relationship between inflammation and ED. If so, non-steroidal anti-inflammatory drugs should help. However, a study done in 2011 at the Department of Urology at Kaiser Permanente's Los Angeles Medical Center found the reverse to be true (Gleason 2010).

A publication in the Journal of Urology found men who take non-steroidal anti-inflammatory drugs three times a day were 2.4 times more likely to have erectile dysfunction compared to men who did not take the medications on a regular basis. If you are taking the over-the-counter equivalent of these medications and are experiencing problems, consult a doctor about possible options, including consumption of natural anti-inflammatory nutritional supplements such as fish oil, turmeric, cinnamon, etc. Anti-inflammatory drug examples include:

- Naproxen (Anaprox, Naprelan, Naprosyn)
- Indomethacin (Indocin)

Parkinson's Disease Medications

While it is possible to live a long happy life after being diagnosed with Parkinson's Disease, people with this condition will likely have to address issues relating to sexual function. Erectile dysfunction and other forms of sexual dysfunction can be the result of the disease itself and the medications used to treat other disease symptoms. Between sixty percent and eighty percent of all men and women diagnosed with Parkinson's report sexual difficulties. The number of young Parkinson's patients reporting difficulty is calculated at thirty percent compared to three percent to fifteen percent of healthy individuals in the same age range (**www.webmd.com**).

The disease can impact sexual functions as a result of damage to central dopamine pathways or by lowering testosterone and estrogen levels. Additionally, some Parkinson's medications can impact sexual function, including the following:

- Biperiden (Akineton)
- Benztropine (Cogentin)
- Trihexyphenidyl (Artane)
- Procyclidine (Kemadrin)
- Bromocriptine (Parlodel)
- Levodopa (Sinemet)

Identifying the source of your sexual difficulties can be important if you have been diagnosed with Parkinson's Disease. But the most important thing is to discuss options with your doctor. While you might not be able to change your condition or your medication, other prescriptions or plans can help address this issue in patients of all ages.

Antiarrythmics

These medications are prescribed to treat abnormal heart rhythms that result from irregular electrical activity of the heart. Several medications used to treat this condition have been known to interfere with sexual performance, including:

- Flecainide (Tambocor)
- Procainamide (Procanbid)
- Amiodarone (Cardarone)
- Soltalol (Betapace)
- Disopyramide (Norpace)
- Metoprolol or Troprol (Beta Blockers)
- Calan (Calcium Channel Blockers)

Muscle Relaxants

A man's ability to achieve and sustain an erection is dependent on the healthy operation of a network of systems that causes vascular tissue to fill with blood. Erectile dysfunction occurs when the body experiences a breakdown anywhere in the sequence of events that lead to an erection. Since there are several muscles involved in obtaining and maintaining an erection and orgasm, muscle relaxers can serve as a breakdown in this sequence.

Since muscle relaxers can be important for men in maintaining other aspects of health, including treatment of pain or injury, consider engaging in sexual activity prior to taking these medications. Also, your doctor will know of a muscle relaxer less known to have sexual side effects. Two prescribed drugs that are commonly listed as causing erectile dysfunction are:

- Cyclobenzaprine (Flexeril)
- Orphenadrine (Norflex)

Prostate Cancer Medications/Chemotherapy Drugs

Both the surgery to remove prostate cancer and the medicines used to treat the condition can lead to erectile problems. When a doctor removes prostate (and bladder) cancer, often the surgeon must remove nerves and tissues surrounding the affected areas. The result can be temporary or even permanent erectile dysfunction. Radiation therapy used to treat prostate cancer can also lead to sexual side-effects.

In addition to surgery and radiation, medications and chemotherapy drugs can lead to ED. Some examples include:

- Flutamide (Eulexin)
- Leuprolide (Lupron)
- Busulfan (Myleran)
- Cyclophosphamide (Cytoxan)

Once in remission, sexual complications associated with drug treatments should clear. However, if sexual dysfunction persists, it would be wise to consult a doctor regarding any damage that might have occurred during surgery or radiation and what can be done to correct such issues.

PRP injected into the surgical area can facilitate the regeneration of nervous tissue, and new blood supply. This regeneration has been found to reverse erectile dysfunction in rats who have undergone similar tissue injury (2009 — PRP applied to perineum post "crush injury" to simulate radical prostatectomy: **www.ncbi.nlm.nih.gov/pubmed/19151738**. 2012 — The Neuroprotective Effect of Platelet-rich Plasma on Erectile Function in Bilateral Cavernous Nerve Injury Rat Model: **www.jsm.jsexmed.org/article/S1743-6095%2815%2933795-4/pdf**. 2013 — Finally asking the question about "optimized PRP" and realizing better results: **www.ncbi.nlm.nih.gov/pubmed/23950105**).

Many physicians are using the Priapus Shot™ to help men recover sexual function post prostate surgery. It is my opinion that PRP injections after prostate surgery will be standard of care in the not so distant future, much the way the use of PRP post heart surgery and plastic surgery is used to facilitate healing.

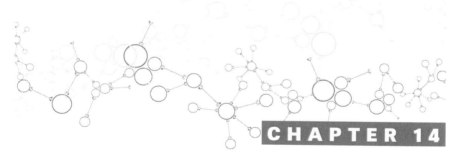

CHAPTER 14

Subtle Changes and Large Events Can Both Cause Changes in Sexual Function

While the previous chapters covered some of the leading causes of sexual dysfunction, there are several other events or factors that can lead to temporary or long-term sexual problems for both sexes. These factors can be as large as life-altering events like heart attacks or trauma and are as easy-to-correct as diet and habits.

I am sure it will come as little surprise that a major event such as a stroke can impact a person's sexual wellness, but you might be surprised to learn that smoking and drinking alcohol have a negative impact as well.

Heart Attacks and Strokes

Studies show that sexual dissatisfaction is common in both male and female stroke patients and those recovering from a heart attack. Both psychological and social factors effect sexual function and quality of life.

Interestingly, studies show that 57 percent of stroke patients report a decrease in sexual interest and their partners reported a sixty-five percent decrease in libido after the episode. This likely means that the libido changes are more psychological than physical. A good sex therapist or couple's counselor should be added to the team to help couples address psychological issues and fears that may be affecting a healthy activity level.

Patients recovering from heart disease face similar issues. The fear of knowing if the patient can handle sexual activity or not is constant. According to the American Heart Association, it is probably safe to have sex if the patient's cardiovascular disease has been stabilized. In fact, conditions such as heart attacks rarely occur during sexual activity so there is little reason to wait to become sexual active again. The health benefits of an intimate relationship far out weight the risks.

If a patient or their partner is finding it difficult to have sex after a heart attack or stroke, an open question and answer session with a physician will probably help alleviate concerns. If the patient experiences prolonged sexual problems such as erectile dysfunction, it might be a good idea for them to be evaluated for other potential causes. There are many options for treatment and full recovery of sexual satisfaction.

The need for a skilled sex therapist cannot be understated when big life changes in health occur. Medical doctors can be poorly equipped to address and treat these "real" issues.

Surgeries (Prostate and Bladder)

At times, the surgical procedure needed to address prostate and bladder cancer can cause damage by removing tissue and nerves in the pelvic region. Rarely, it is necessary to cut or remove nerves that control penile blood flow. While these nerves are not responsible for orgasm, they can cause issues with erectile function. Radiation therapy can also cause damage to this area and result in various degrees of sexual complications.

New nerve-sparing techniques aimed at lowering the incidence of impotence are being developed and used in these surgeries, which should improve results dramatically. Temporary impotence is also associated with these procedures, even when new surgical techniques are used.

There are rat studies that illustrate the benefit of PRP injection and daily penile pumping to completely restore erectile function after nerve damage. Intracavernosal Pharmacology (ICP) three times a week in conjunction with PRP injection will likely have similar benefits in humans.

Physical Trauma/Herniated Lumbar Disc

Trauma to the pelvic region or spinal cord can cause damage to the veins and nerves needed to achieve and maintain erection. In fact, any injury to the pelvis, bladder, spinal cord, and penis can cause sexual complications for men making it difficult to achieve orgasms.

Physical trauma or injuries can cause a venous leak- a condition where the veins in the penis do not constrict properly resulting in impotence.

Neurological Conditions

Spinal cord and brain injuries can cause impotence when they interrupt the transfer of nerve impulses from the brain to the penis. Other nerve disorders that can negatively impact sexual functions include Multiple Sclerosis, Parkinson's disease, and Alzheimer's disease.

Recreational Chemical Consumption

The use of tobacco, alcohol, and/or illegal substances can damage vessels, making it difficult for blood to reach the penis in order to fulfill an erection. Smoking in particular hardens arteries and dramatically increases a man's risk of erectile dysfunction. Not surprising, there are more than 200 prescribed drugs that report negative sexual side effects (**www.webmd.com**).

Smoking and use of alcohol (and illegal substances) can have a severe effect on breathing, kidney processes, hormone production, neurotransmitter balance and blood flow. There are many conditions that impact sexual wellness and blood flow is perhaps one of the most important factors. Anything that causes your blood to clog will eventually lead to a heart attack or stroke and impair sexual function. In fact, sexual dysfunction might be an early sign of danger for one of these events.

Nutrient Deficiencies

A poor diet can lead to negative health consequences, so it should not be surprising that an unhealthy diet contributes to an unhealthy sex life. In particular, when blood flow is compromised to a man or woman's pelvic area, sexual dysfunction can occur.

A study published in the Journal of Sexual Medicine found that atherosclerosis of the arterial bed supplying female pelvic anatomy can lead to decreased vaginal engorgement and clitoral erectile insufficiency syndrome which can lead to female sexual dysfunction (Esposito 2009).

Researchers found women with high cholesterol levels reported significantly lower instances of arousal, orgasm, lubrication, and satisfaction than their healthy counterparts. Therefore, it is reasonable to conclude that a healthy diet that helps lower cholesterol levels, blood sugar and blood pressure will prove beneficial to men and women and their individual sexual functions. There are also several vitamins that are beneficial and include the following:

Vitamin A

Vitamin A is important for testosterone production throughout male life. Early in life, a vitamin A deficiency can even delay puberty in boys. Consumption of this vitamin can help a man boost his testosterone levels while considering his best treatment options for Low-T.

Vitamin E

Sometimes called the "sex vitamin," Vitamin E protects sex hormones from degradation by free radicals and is necessary for the healthy production of sperm (and sperm motility).

Zinc/Magnesium/Selenium

These three minerals are important in sexual function. Zinc supplements can reverse sexual dysfunction in men undergoing renal dialysis. Low magnesium levels are attributed to problems with premature ejaculation caused by vasoconstriction in the penis.

Selenium supplementation has been found to increase testosterone levels while improving sperm count and mobility.

These minerals keep the body running in an optimal environment. Even the most subtle deficiencies can interfere with optimal physical and emotional function in both men and women.

Amino Acids, Arginine

Amino Acids and Arginine are essential in producing nitric acid, which acts as powerful vasodilators and play a critical role in initiating and maintaining an erection. Trial research indicates that nutrient-rich, whole foods with nutritional supplements can ensure good health for men and a solid sex life.

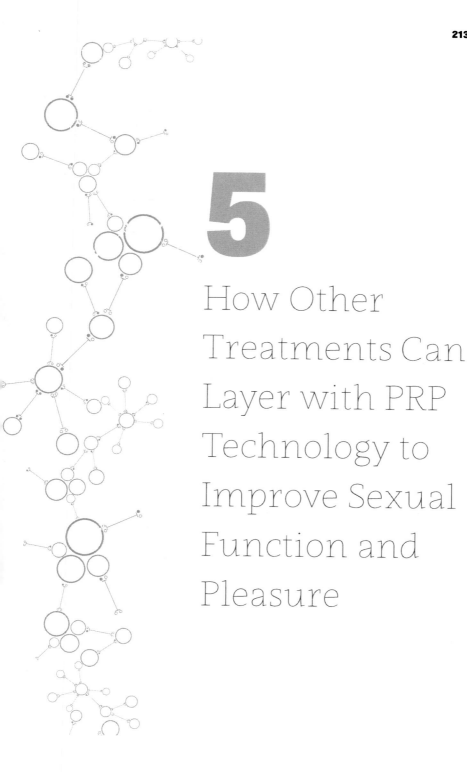

5

How Other Treatments Can Layer with PRP Technology to Improve Sexual Function and Pleasure

This section details how PRP enhances medical treatments, specifically sexual dysfunction therapy and urinary incontinence. PRP can augment and improve results; it works synergistically complimenting other treatments without negative interactions.

First, I'll layout several treatment possibilities and present the pros and cons for each option. In my practice, there's strong focus on tailoring treatments that are designed for each patient; alternatives that are less invasive and more successful than others.

Second, I'll examine how PRP works to improve some of the treatments. This is an area of medicine that will produce significant benefits for men and women in their relationships, quality of life, and general happiness in the decades to come. It's exciting to think of the possibilities that PRP holds as a preventative and regenerative solution.

CHAPTER 15

Why Men and Women Both Need "Optimal" Hormone Levels and Not Just "Normal" Hormone Levels: How and Why to Restore Hormone Balance

As you've read, hormone levels and biochemistry change in men and women as they age. I recommend the use of bio-identical hormones (BHRT) as opposed to non-bio-identical hormones (HRT). Not all hormone treatments are the same. In fact, both men and women need *optimal* levels of hormones; some of which they might not realize they possess.

What Are Hormones & Why Do They Decline?

Simply put, hormones are the body's messengers that transport information from the brain to the glands, from the glands to the cells, and from the cells to the brain. Hormones also rejuvenate, regenerate and restore our bodies. In fact, hormones are so vital that diet and exercise alone will not achieve maximum benefit if there's an imbalance.

Hormones enable the physiological changes that happen in our bodies as we move from childhood through adolescents and into adulthood. They are at their highest levels from ages 25-30, the same period when the body is at its strongest and healthiest. From that point on, hormones decline each year.

Physicians were taught that as we age, our hormones decline. It is now becoming clear that as our hormones decline, we age! So why does this fact matter and what can you do about it?

Thanks to scientific and medical advancements, we are living longer — on average — than ever before. Our advances in healthcare, vaccinations, sanitation and food preservatives have drastically increased our life spans. But the glands that produce our hormones have not caught up to our scientific achievements and they do not regenerate after a certain age. In fact, these glands continue to decline, producing fewer hormones with each passing year.

As we age, it becomes increasingly important for both men and women to keep their hormones balanced to protect against fatigue, mood swings, disease, obesity, bone loss, muscle loss, brain degeneration, immune system malfunction, and to enjoy an over-all healthier sense of well-being.

Natural Hormones vs. Synthetic Hormones

Not all hormone therapies are created equally. Synthetic hor-mones, like Provera or Premarin are derived from plant pro-gesterone and animal estrogens. They are chemicals that act as toxins in the body. Because they are not natural, the body cannot metabolize them properly. These are the hormone treatments that have been linked with cancer and yet, still prescribed regularly by physicians today. **I use only use natural bio-identical hormones.** Unlike synthetic hormones, bio-identical hormones or natu-ral hormones are replicas of the body's own natural hormones. They're made from soy, yams and other plant extracts, which are converted to be biologically identical to the same hormones the body produces. As a result, the body recognizes and metabolizes them normally and predictably.

For optimal safety and results, replace only hormones that are low. Evaluate symptoms and retest hormone levels regularly to be sure that optimal ranges and ratios are maintained. It is important to note that this medical "art" relies more on experience than it does lab values. It's not uncommon for me to treat a patient and not the numbers when the numbers do not seem to correlate with the symptoms.

What Do Hormones Do and Which Ones Do We Need?

Teenagers often display emotional and physical changes attributed to hormones. There's definitely a surge at this age and we see it in temper spikes and outbursts of tears. Here's an explanation of these hormones and why we need them, especially at ages 15, 25, 55, and beyond.

HUMAN GROWTH HORMONE — the growth hormone

- Decreases body fat
- Increases muscle mass
- Improves tissue healing and protein synthesis
- Increases bone density
- Quicker illness recovery
- Increases capacity to exercise
- Increases skin hydration and elasticity
- Improves sense of well being
- Decreases incidence of illness

TESTOSTERONE — the "male" hormone that is LARGELY overlooked in women

- Improves brain function, concentration and mood
- Increases energy and stamina; both physical and mental
- Increases strength and improves muscle recoveryIncreases bone density
- Increases libido

- Improves sexual sensitivity
- Improves sexual function
- Improves HDL and LDL levels
- Improves cardiovascular health

DHEA — the mother of hormones

- Improves neurological function
- Increases sense of well being
- Improves immune function
- Improves stress tolerance
- Increases metabolism

ESTROGENS — the "stimulating" hormone

- Accelerates metabolism
- Protects against heart disease, stroke
- Decreases cholesterol — Increase HDL and lowers LDL
- Increases vaginal lubrication
- Thickens the vaginal wall
- Lowers incidence of Alzheimer's
- Increases bone formation
- Improves memory
- Promotes sexual receptivity
- Alleviates symptoms of menopause: headaches, mood swings, bloating, hot flashes, fatigue, waning libido

- Anti-inflammatory properties
- Testosterone can only improve libido in the presence of estrogen
- Maintains collagen integrity and regeneration for healthy skin, joint and tendons

PROGESTERONE — the "feel good" hormone

- Protects against breast and uterine cancer
- Protects against fibrocystic disease
- Helps fat metabolism
- Helps normalize blood sugar
- Helps reverse osteoporosis
- Helps thyroid hormone function
- Acts as a natural antidepressant
- Protects against nervousness
- Protects against anxiety and irritability
- Sensitizes the cells to estrogen
- Enhances the function of serotonin in the brain
- Regulates immune response and acts as an anti-inflammatory agent

PREGNENELONE — the gateway hormone

- Promotes formation of other hormones
- Repairs brain and nerve tissue

- Enhances many brain functions
- Reduces aging skin
- Improves sense of well being
- Increases energy and mobility
- Improves sleep quality
- Reduces harmful stress effects
- Reduces aging brain deficiencies

THYROID — the hormone of metabolism

- Has an effect on every cell of the body.
- Modulates energy production and metabolic rate
- Involved in protein synthesis
- Works synergistically with growth hormone
- Essential to proper development and differentiation of all cells
- Regulates protein, fat, and carbohydrate metabolism
- Regulates body temperature
- Regulates heart rate
- Plays a role in controlling appetite

INSULIN — the hormone of storage

- Responsible for getting blood sugar into all cells
- Increases fat storage
- Increases risk of diabetes, hypertension, and stroke

MELATONIN — the hormone of sleep

- Powerful antioxidant that crosses the blood brain barrier
- Anti-inflammatory effects
- Delays neurodegenerative process of aging
- Responsible for maintaining sleep cycle
- Prevents migraine headaches
- Improves metabolism
- Helps alleviate "jet-lag"
- Improves mood
- Improves the immune system (by decreasing cortisol)
- Aromatase Inhibitor

CORTISOL — the hormone of stress

- Responsible for responding to stress
- Helps protect against environment (allergens)
- Mobilizes energy, improves fatigue
- Increases appetite for sugar
- Decreases bone mass, muscle mass, and slows down metabolism

Hormones and hormone balance are very important at any age. I prioritize getting my patients balanced when they seek help for fatigue, weight gain, difficulty managing stress, sleep disturbance, decreased libido, sexual dysfunction, and decrease feeling of well-being.

Bio-Identical Hormones (BHRT)

Both bio-identical hormones and non-bio-identical hormones (sometimes called synthetic hormones) are used to alleviate symptoms of hormonal imbalance, but BHRT unlike non bio-identical hormone therapy is also used to correct the hormonal imbalance causing the symptoms. The scientific innovation behind bio-identical hormones is that they are an exact copy of the hormones naturally made by your body and are fully recognized when introduced.

Bio-identical hormones are easy to measure when administering the treatment though creams, capsules, injectable's, sublingual's and pellets. A balance of these hormones will improve the body's function, health, and vitality.

In contrast, non-bioidentical (synthetic) hormones are slightly different molecules from what your body naturally produces. However, that slight difference can generate a very different response by the body. The connections made to medical risks such as cancers are associated with these types of hormone treatments.

It can be easy to confuse the use of BHRT and HRT treatments because even doctors often use the words interchangeably, just as the words Progesterone and Progestin. However, these substances are very different: one is a natural substance while the other is a synthetic creation. Greater wellness is achieved by self-healing (PRP) and introducing substances into the body that are copies of what already exists (BHRT).

When BHRT is administered, the skilled physician can check hormone levels via blood, urine or saliva. Non bio-identical (HRT) levels cannot be measured. Symptoms are effectively treated by both HRT and BHRT but hormone balance is only achieved by BHRT.

Individuals who have experienced symptoms of hormone imbalance should consult their doctors about BHRT. The treatment is successful -even in premenopausal women and younger men. However, before you receive treatment, make sure your health care provider is trained in the evaluation and treatment of hormone imbalances using BHRT.

Cancer is the number one reason why women do not seek hormone replacement therapy and the reason why many doctors are fearful to offer it to patients. It's sad, because patient health and quality of life is likely hindered by this decision. Breast cancer has been prevented by several BHRT treatments. Therefore, it is important for the public to realize that options exist and hormone therapy generally does not result in cancer if the proper treatment procedures are used. In fact, some hormone treatments are protective against cancers, osteoporosis, heart disease, Alzheimer's, and depression.

For over 100 years, the medical community thought that testosterone therapy caused prostate cancer. There were many thousands of men denied treatment who would have benefited. It is now very clear that testosterone therapy does NOT cause cancer, yet still many physicians are not yet on board with this evolving opinion.

Occasionally, poorly conducted studies sponsored by groups with ulterior motives are publicized and sensationalized. This further separates potential patients who would benefit from healthy and life changing hormonal therapies.

Natural progesterone given to balance estrogen has been shown to protect against uterine cancer, breast cancer, and cardiovascular disease. It is synthetic progestin that has been tied to an increase in breast cancer and cardiovascular disease.

Whether or not you seek BHRT or HRT, hormone imbalance itself could prove more dangerous than the associated cancer risk. I cannot emphasize enough that BHRT, when prescribed and monitored by an expert, can be safer and better for your overall health and well-being than not pursuing hormone treatment at all.

Hormone Replacement Therapy in Women

There is more than one way to administer hormone treatments and this can impact the benefits women realize from the therapy. I prescribe BHRT exclusively and monitor symptoms and hormone levels regularly in my practice.

Systemic Hormone Therapy

Systemic estrogen is administered as a pill, gel, cream/spray, skin patch, injection and pellet therapy. It is highly effective in decreasing menopausal hot flashes and night sweats, mood swings, headaches, weight gain as well as vaginal dryness, itching, burning, and discomfort during intercourse.

Low-Dose Vaginal Products

Estrogen therapy for vaginal atrophy, dryness and urinary symptoms is a localized treatment that is packaged as a vaginal ring, cream, suppositories, oils or tablet. Among other health benefits, this therapy enriches sexual function by enhancing vaginal tone and elasticity, increasing vaginal blood flow, and improving lubrication. At times, estrogen is combined with a second hormone to improve the benefits women experience. I will often compound all BHRT hormones into one vaginal cream to administer systemic benefit and additional vaginal health.

Estrogen and Progesterone Medications

I prescribe progesterone (a bio-identical hormone) to balance estrogen treatments. Optimal natural Progesterone levels have been associated with decreased breast and uterine cancer risk. It is often taught that if a woman has experienced a hysterectomy, she does not need progesterone treatment. This could not be further from the truth. Women have progesterone receptors in many areas of the body including the brain. Postmenopausal and premenopausal women need the optimal amount of bio-identical progesterone to balance their energy, metabolism, mood and general sense of well-being. Progesterone is necessary in cell signaling to work with the thyroid and also to facilitate blood sugar balance.

The benefits of hormone therapy are evident, but deciding between bio-identical hormone treatments and non bio-identical hormone treatment can mark the different between success and failure for many women. Health risks associated with non bio-identical hormone replacement therapy include breast cancer, heart disease, stroke, and blood clots.

On the other hand, benefits of bio-identical hormone replacement therapy for women include:

- Elimination of symptoms of menopause such as night sweats and hot flashes
- Decreases or elimination of vaginal dryness, burning and itching
- Relieves pain associated with intercourse
- Elevates energy levels and improve mood, memory, and concentration
- Facilitates fat loss and enhanced muscle tone
- Improves sex drive, function and satisfaction
- Smooths skin and strengthens bones
- Reduces the risk of heart disease

Women who experience early menopause (prior to the age of 40) in particular may benefit from hormone treatment. Without estrogen therapy, women who experience premature meno-pause have a higher risk of osteoporosis, coronary heart disease, Parkinson's, dementia, anxiety or depression, and sexual dysfunc-tion. Therefore, women in this category should seek hormone evaluation to make sure that optimal hormone levels and balance are achieved.

Bio identical testosterone is a hormone that is most often un-derutilized in women and always found to be safe and protective against breast cancer. Women need testosterone for metabolism, brain health, bone health, and sexual health. Testosterone helps women to have a healthy libido, physical and mental stamina, mental focus and uplifted general state of well-being. Testosterone can help maintain strength and stability.

Testosterone pellets have been around since the 1930s and found to be safe and effective. Women are treated successfully for migraines and found protected from breast cancer with the use of testosterone and the combined Testosterone and Anastrazole Pellets.

Hormone Replacement Therapy in Men

Andropause is the male version of menopause, though it takes place over a longer period of time and has subtle onsets. Naturally, testosterone levels begin to decrease after the age of 30 at a rate of one percent per year. By the time a man is in his 40's or even 50's, he should consider hormone replacement therapy as much as any woman going through menopause. Hormone balance is required for proper male sexual development and reproductive function, as well as, muscle bulk, red blood cell level, and bone density.

Hormone replacement therapy can help symptoms of low testosterone. The treatment can be given through muscular injections, testosterone patches worn on the body, testosterone gel applied topically and Testosterone Pellet Therapy. The frequency of treatment depends on the form of application used. My preference is Testosterone Pellet Therapy because it closely mimics the physiologic release of hormones than any other treatment vehicle.

Like women, men can use a bio-identical hormone replacement treatment to address their declining levels of testosterone. The science behind BHRT testosterone is that it matches structurally with the hormones produced by the human body and can create the same physiological response. The aim is not to achieve an overdose or supra-physiologic dose of hormones in the man's body, but to bring his testosterone levels up to a point that the man was accustomed to in his younger, healthier years.

Male patients report BHRT benefits that include:

- Improves energy levels and physical and mental endurance
- Increases muscle mass, tone, and fat loss
- Elevates sex drive and enhances performance
- Benefits memory and concentration as well as sleep patterns
- Decreases joint and muscle pain while improving bone strength
- Improves cholesterol levels and protects against heart disease

There are some details to consider when balancing male hormones. Sometimes symptoms of estrogen and testosterone imbalance can occur when starting testosterone therapy in a man. These "side effects" of testosterone treatment are due to aromatase activity and the facilitation of the conversion of testosterone to estradiol. These minor effects include fluid retention, acne, and increased urination or worsening urinary challenges. These effects can be avoided when the proper monitoring and treatment is administered by experience hormone specialist.

More serious side effects can ensue and therefore, hormone levels and treatment strategies should be closely monitored and managed. These more serious effects can include decreased testicle sizes, infertility, decreased sperm count, breast enlargement, sleep apnea, changes in cholesterol, and increased red cell count.

Testosterone may stimulate an already present slow growing prostate cancer. Testosterone does not cause prostate cancer, but PSA is monitored to indicate stability of the prostate tissue throughout treatment. Testosterone therapy often reduces bothersome symptoms of benign prostatic hypertrophy (BPH).

Every man deserves optimal hormone balance. There is new and ongoing evidence that supports testosterone replacement therapy in men who experience symptoms of andropause (hormone decline and imbalance).

ALL men benefit from optimal hormone balance. The trick is to find a physician who understand the "art" of hormone replacement and how to properly customize the treatment. Monitoring hormone levels and other physiologic markers is absolutely necessary to achieve optimal results and improved health and wellness.

"My Favorite Way to Balance Hormones"

Bio-identical Hormone Replacement Pellet Therapy

Data supports that hormone replacement therapy with pellet implants is an effective bio-identical method to deliver hormones in both men and women. Implants, placed under the skin, consistently release small, physiologic doses of hormones.

BHRT Pellet Implant History

Bio-identical hormone pellet implants have been used in the U.S., Europe, and Australia since the 1930s. In fact, pellet implants were a very popular mode of hormone administration in the U.S. until the 1970s, when many oral and topical commercial products were developed. While the demand for pellets diminished in the U.S. until recently, pellet implants continued to be a very popular mode of hormone administration throughout Europe and Australia.

Over 70 years of research has illustrated the benefits of pellet implants in administering hormones in both women and men.

- Pellet implants deliver consistent, physiologic levels of hormones.

- The consistent and physiologic dosing has been shown to maintain and improve bone density.

- Pellet implants bypass the liver and don't negatively impact clotting factors and the risk of blood clots, elevated blood pressure, lipid levels, glucose, or liver function.

Pellet implants have consistently been shown to improve:

- Cardiovascular health

- Sex drive and libido
- Headaches and migraines
- Insomnia
- Hot flashes and night sweats
- Anxiety, irritability and depression
- Muscle and joint aches and pains
- Bone density
- Mood
- Endometriosis and uterine fibroids
- Fatigue
- Urinary incontinence
- Vaginal dryness

Pellet implants are compounded using biologically identical hormones (most often Estradiol and Testosterone and recently a combination of Testosterone and Anastrazole). The hormones are pressed/fused into very small cylinders about the size of a grain of rice. There is an FDA approved 75mg pellet marketed as Testopel.

Pellet insertion is a very simple in-office procedure done under local anesthesia. The pellets are inserted subcutaneously (under the fatty lining of skin), either in the lower abdomen, the upper buttock or flank (love handle) through a very small incision. The incision is closed with surgical glue or sterile-tape strips. Implants placed under the skin consistently release small, physiologic doses of hormones.

Pellet Implants typically last between 3-5 months, depending on how rapidly the hormones are metabolized. Some patients begin to feel symptom relief within 48 hours, while others may take up to two weeks to notice a marked difference. The pellets do not need to be removed. They are completely dissolved by the body.

Generally, there are minimal side-effects associated with the pellet implantation procedure. Complications include: minor bleeding, bruising, infection, and pellet extrusion. Other than slight bruising, the other complications are very rare. Hormone side-effects vary and should be discussed with your hormone specialist.

Based on existing hormone levels and health history, the practitioner will make a hormone replacement recommendation. Once pellets have been inserted, hormone levels will be reevaluated prior to the insertion of the next round of pellets or other form of hormone delivery. After the first year of pellet therapy, the practitioner may suggest testing less frequently based upon patient feedback and prior hormone levels.

Hormone levels will be evaluated via lab testing before therapy is started to establish baseline levels. Labs should include a FSH, LH, Prolactin, estradiol, total and free testosterone, TSH, free T3, and free T4. Men need a PSA, sensitive estradiol, free and total testosterone, complete metabolic panel, and complete blood count prior to starting therapy. Thyroid hormone levels may also be evaluated. Levels will be reevaluated during hormone therapy, usually prior to insertion of the next set of pellets.

Pellet dosing for both men and women is based on patient weight, symptoms, age, activity, and hormone levels. Adjustments are made as the dose is calibrated to optimal levels of effect, balancing lab findings, patient response and side effects. Women will typically receive between 50 and 170mg every 3-5 months, where men receive between 1000-2000mg every 4-6 months.

In women, blood levels of total testosterone at peak (4-6 weeks post pellet implantation) will commonly increase to between 200-500ng/dL and return to upper end of normal endogenous levels when symptoms return and pellet implantation is due. This drop typically happens in 3-4 months as blood levels decrease, but can be avoided by adjusting the pellet implantation frequency.

In men, blood levels of total testosterone at peak are expected to rise between 800-1200ng/dL and drop to 400-600 ng/dL when symptoms return. This drop typically happens in 3-4 months as blood levels decrease, but can be avoided by adjusting the pellet implantation frequency.

Remarkably, Testosterone Pellet Therapy in women has clearly been shown NOT to increase the risk of breast cancer or breast cancer recurrence but to actually decrease the risk. In fact, testosterone pellets and testosterone combined with Anastrazole in pellets are being shown in clinical study to reduce the risk of breast cancer and as a treatment for women with metastatic breast cancer.

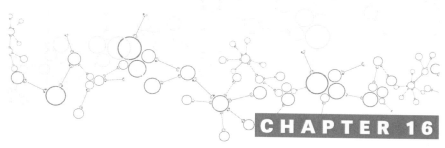

CHAPTER 16

Why Do Men Grow Breasts and Women Grow Mustaches? How Men and Women are Hormonally Similar and What Happens When the Balance is Tipped in the Wrong Direction

There's quite a bit of talk and advertisements concerning Low-T treatments for men. However, testosterone is not the only hormone level that changes. Just as women need estrogen and testosterone, men also require both hormones. As men age and testosterone declines, their estrogen levels increase, further interfering with optimal function.

It is that increase in estrogen that causes men to become more effeminate as they age. Men in their 60's or 70's who maintain good muscle tone and body mass, probably are on some kind of hormone therapy.

Hormone imbalance significantly affects the quality of life. The following changes were cited in the 2006 review article "Testosterone and men's quality of life" by Ignacio Moncada:

- Energy
- Emotional functioning
- Social functioning
- Social emotional
- Mental functioning
- Physical functioning
- Sexual functioning

Conversely, women experience variances in their hormone levels that cause them to become less feminine as they age. Changes can result in an increase in facial hair and decreases in the quality of skin, nails, and/or hair.

Balancing hormones isn't just a matter of raising estrogen and lowering testosterone. A woman needs testosterone for bone health, brain health, metabolism, sense of well-being and sexual health. Therefore, achieving a balance that allows a woman to maintain her femininity while optimizing sex drive is a matter of carefully measuring, correcting, and monitoring all hormone levels.

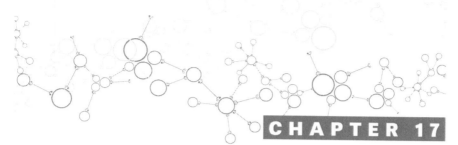

CHAPTER 17

How Nutrition and Supplements Make a Difference in Enhancing Sexual Function and Experience

While the production of hormones in men and women are paramount for sexual function, there are several other treatment strategies that can be used instead of — or in conjunction with — hormone replacement treatment. These treatments plans range from natural (healthy habits and nutrition) to mechanical tools (penile pumps or vacuum devices).

Optimal Health & Nutrition

A healthy lifestyle balances the physical, mental and sexual conditions of the body. My patients are advised to choose whole fresh food, clean filtered water, purposeful regular movements, deep breathing, and restorative sleep. All are critical to achieve uninhibited sexual response that is essential for maintaining a quality life.

I realize that fitness and diet products are advertised abundantly in our society and that you likely know that a healthy diet supports optimal functionality and an improved body. But it's important to emphasize the relevance proper nutrition is for maintaining good body chemistry and health. A great diet can help prevent cardiovascular disease, high cholesterol, high blood pressure, and diabetes, and lower the chances of experiencing sexual dysfunction caused by these diseases.

Healthy diets consisting of fruits, vegetables, lean proteins, nuts, and oils facilitate energy production, neurotransmitter balance, hormone production, and facilitate all biochemical reactions of the body. You ARE what you eat because it is the molecules of food that run the human machine. Processed food is bad information to the body much like poor quality gas is to your automobile engine. Sure, the engine will run with bad gas but the performance is significantly affected.

I make my living helping people who are not functioning optimally; physically, mentally, and sexually. Poor quality food will lead to deterioration of all bodily systems. Whole fresh foods will reverse this deterioration and contribute to wellness that is obvious to all.

Furthermore, a woman maintaining a healthy weight and exercise regimen can help counter issues she experiences during and post-menopause. This is important to helping a woman maintain a positive body-image and self-confidence which is a large part of her sexual experience.

Besides healthy eating and exercise, an individual will realize their greatest health and sexual experience by limiting alcohol, eliminating processed foods and artificial sweeteners and by not smoking. While many people probably think alcohol leads to sex rather than preventing it, drinking has been known to hinder sexual responsiveness, function and satisfaction. So alcohol might lower inhibition, but it can also decrease sexual pleasure. Smoking restricts blood flow to sexual organs and decreases sexual arousal as a result (**www.webmd.com**).

Nutritional Guide for Men & Women

As an added bonus for readers, I've included a link to my Studio Solution 4-Phase Program at the end of this book. This program uses food and exercise as a prescription to influence your metabolism, restore balance, and to reduce the risk of developing cancer, diabetes and cardiovascular disease.

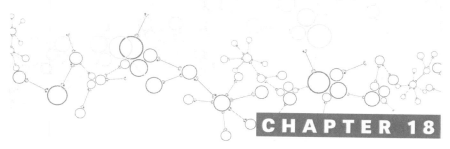

CHAPTER 18

Is the "Little Blue Pill" All There Is?

When Viagra came on the market, many people thought, "Great, problem solved!" But Viagra does not work for everyone and there are many other options available. This chapter is dedicated to exploring a wide-range of treatments to improve sexual well-being with or without the use of PRP therapy. Though I must emphasize, that any and all of these could prove more effective when combined with PRP treatments.

Oral Drug Treatments

The Viagra wave has been fairly prolific and the advertising of competing products, such as Levitra or Cialis, have captured the market share, as well. All medications in this segment work to improve erectile function by increasing nitric oxide, a naturally produced chemical in the body. When the chemical goes into effect, it opens and relaxes blood vessels in the penis, helping the man achieve and maintain an erection.

PRP treatment (Priapus Shot™) regenerates penile tissue and therefore improves the potential for oral medications to work in men where they previously didn't and also to improve efficacy of the medication.

It is important to mention that oral medications do not work on their own, meaning that if a man takes a pill, he will not induce an erection without sexual stimulation. So, many men are fearful of medications because of the unknown. They are most often too embarrassed to ask enough questions to fully educate themselves on the treatments that are available. And, far too many doctors don't have the knowledge of the treatment options — or they don't take the time to probe into the subject of the patient's sexual function in order to know when and which treatment is warranted.

At times, these medications can be unhealthy for a man with certain conditions. If he has heart problems, blood pressure issues, a history of stroke, eye problems, or liver/kidney disease, he should consult with a doctor first.

Even those healthy enough to take erectile dysfunction medicine, the side effects are plenty: headaches, indigestion, stuffy/runny nose, muscle aches, vision changes, or dizziness/faintness. A more serious side effect that has proven a source for comedies is the erection that does not go away on its own. This is a rare condition called priapism that I mentioned earlier and requires medical treatment to avoid damage to the penis.

In recent years, pharmaceutical research has found a potential answer to the request for a "female Viagra." In 2010, ABC News reported that the US Food and Drug Administration (FDA) was considering approval of Flibanserin, an oral drug showing potential benefits in enhancing women's sex lives (**www.abcnews.com**). Dr. Marie Savard, a "Good Morning America" medical contributor, said that flibanserisn works on a woman's brain chemistry to increase her desire for sex (Clarke 2010).

Studies of the drug focused on pre-menopausal women and showed an increase on the number of satisfying sexual experiences from 2.7 to 4.5 per month. The drug was declined by the FDA in 2010, but in June of 2013, Sprout Pharmaceuticals confirmed they had resubmitted the drug for FDA approval (**www.news-medical. net**) as a treatment for Hypoactive Sexual Desire Disorder (HSDD) in pre-menopausal women. In 2015 under pressure, the FDA approved the drug under the trade name Addyi. January 27, 2016, the FDA released a statement that brought to light little benefit and significant risk.

Another medication that has proven successful in helping women enjoy more sexual pleasure is Osphena, a non-estrogen oral pill that improves certain physical changes of the vagina and significantly relieves moderate to server painful intercourse in menopausal women (**www.osphena.com**).

Osphena has been used by women to make vaginal tissue thicker and less fragile, which can help with sexual pleasure. Common side effects include hot flashes, vaginal discharge, muscle spasms, and increased sweating. More severe — but rare — side effects can include stroke, blood clots, and cancer of the uterus lining.

If a woman has experienced vaginal bleeding or has a medical history with blood clots, stroke, heart attack, or liver problems, she should probably not take Osphena. A discussion with your medical provider concerning your entire medical history is vital to deciding if Osphena or Osphena with estrogen treatments are right for you.

I am not in a hurry to prescribe the new drug "Osphena" since there is little long term data and potential serious side effects. The O-Shot™ done by administering the patient's own platelet rich plasma offers regenerative benefit with little to no side effects. PRP and bio-identical hormone optimization has been effective for most women in my practice at restoring sexual desire, sexual pleasure, and sexual performance.

The PRP and BHRT combination also has many systemic benefits that I feel women deserve. It is important to understand the cause of the symptoms of imbalance and when possible to correct the imbalances rather than to simply add a chemical to treat the symptoms.

I am NOT a purist by any means, and I don't want you to think that I am judging any of the medications for sexual dysfunction as "bad," but I do feel strongly that the focus should be to repair the "foundation" when possible with BHRT, optimal nutrition and regenerative procedures such as O Shot™ and Priapus Shot™ before considering chemical symptom relief as a treatment.

The goal for my own life and the lives of my patients is happiness and satisfaction. I am a proponent for "whatever it takes" to accomplish this end. Of course, a very careful exploration and discussion of risks and benefits is absolutely necessary before starting any form of therapy.

As a side note, there is a specific hormone treatment I do prescribe to my female patients that can help with libido, orgasm and sexual satisfaction. Oxytocin is known for playing a key role in maternal bonding and lactation, but it also is vital to women achieving orgasm, pair bonding, dealing with anxiety, and addressing mood disorders (Hurlemann 2010). For this reason, I have found it to be a positive medication to prescribe.

Creams & Gels

If a woman is experiencing vaginal irritation, dryness, or discomfort, it is recommended that she make a few changes to personal habits; using clean water for washing the vagina, using only white unscented toilet paper, and washing underwear in dye-free/perfume-free detergents. Also, she should avoid using lotions and perfumed products on her inner vulva.

There are several over-the-counter/non-medicated vaginal lubricants available as well as prescription-only topical forms of bio-identical estrogen, DHEA and testosterone therapy. Vaginal lubricants come in liquid and gel form and are applied directly to the vagina and vulva (or a partner's penis) prior to sexual intercourse. Lubricants provide temporary relief for dryness and other painful issues that can occur during sex, but can sometimes add to the long term problem since they are often alcohol based.

In hormonally imbalanced women, vaginal estrogen, and testosterone products deliver hormone directly to the vaginal tissue to stimulate repair and regeneration of thin fragile hormone deprived vaginal tissue. This treatment has proven to restore vaginal blood flow and improve tissue thickness and elasticity. Vaginal creams can be applied in small doses a couple of times a week. They should not be used prior to intercourse so they are not absorbed through a partner's skin.

Moisturizers are another option to improve sexual comfort, and they differ from lubricants in a few ways. They are absorbed into the skin and cling to the vaginal lining in order to copy natural secretions. They are applied regularly rather than just before sex, so that they produce benefits that last several days. They can be used in connection with lubricants if it improves sexual comfort (**www.menopause.org**).

A wide range of lubricants are available as water-based or silicone-based products, but I have found that the best sexual lubricant is extra virgin coconut oil. Natural coconut oil is nourishing to the vaginal tissues and to the penis. Coconut oils lasts longer, tastes great and is non-toxic. There are rarely allergic reactions to this natural product.

Injections

Intracavernosal Pharmacology (ICP) is an old treatment therapy that has a great deal of utility. ICP is comprised of various combinations of medications that are injected with a very small needle into the side of the penis when erection is desired. **This treatment**

rarely fails. The medications injected are vasodilators. They cause a significant increase in blood flow to the penis resulting in a robust erection. The needle is tiny and the injection is virtually painless especially when an auto-injector is used.

The problem with ICP as I see it is that most of the time, there is a lack of proper customization of the medication as well as incomplete patient education. This lack of detail causes many men to "fail" ICP therapy, thus missing out on the possibility of reliable erection and even possible rehabilitation. ICP is a reliable treatment that I hope make more palatable to men by properly educating them on how best to use it safely and effectively. I think that most men and even most doctors do not understand ICP and therefore are in fear of the consequence of improper use.

ICP when customized appropriately is very safe, reliable and always effective. When not customized or provided to a patient with little understanding, ICP can be a disaster, leading to significant complications and even penis amputation.

The proper way to prescribe ICP is to first provide the patient with a thorough evaluation, starting with a physical examination, penile Doppler to assess blood flow to the penis, a biothesiometer to determine the level of penile sensitivity, age and state of health are also considered. There is a reliable algorhythm that is followed to determine the proper combination of medications and dose of ICP. Once the proper medication is determined, a "trial" injection is administered in the office under physician supervision. This mean that the man is injected in the office with the goal of causing a seventy percent non-sexually stimulated erection. The

ICP injection in the office is a very important part of the diagnostic procedure. Peak blood flow is determined once an erection is achieved.

ICP is warranted in all patient evaluations even if ED is not acknowledged and the primary complaint is premature ejaculation (PE). In fact, ICP can be very effective for a man who suffers from PE because it allows him to ejaculate and yet still maintain an erection to complete the sexual act and to satisfy his partner. The advantage of ICP over oral treatments is that there is no systemic distribution. Gaining control over his ejaculation over a period of time is more realistic since he will often become desensitized to the point when ICP may no longer be necessary, thus the "rehabilitation" that I have been promising. The reliability of a quality erection facilitated by ICP that continues after ejaculation relieves the debilitating anxiety that a man with PE experiences. This "performance anxiety" always makes PE worse since anxiety is an erection killer! Men will often avoid sex and will become embarrassed, depressed, and withdrawn as a result of unsuccessful treatment of PE. PE and ED are both progressive diseases. Progressive meaning that they get worse if not treated aggressively and effectively. PE will often lead to ED.

Once the evaluation is complete, proper quality of erection has been achieved and doses have been determined, the patient is then taught how and when to use the medication at home. Proper patient education and medication customization is essential to success. Proper physician follow-up ensures success since it is very rare that ED and PE cannot be successfully treated.

You can imagine how ICP is a valuable tool to rehabilitation and the eventual reversal of ED and PE in many men. For therapeutic purposes, men should be counseled to use ICP two or three times a week for a duration of 6-12 months. Use "as needed" can be effective but loses its therapeutic value if less than two or three times per week. ICP is part of a complete rehabilitation program and provides men with full control over erection timing, duration and quality.

By facilitating a robust erection with ICP, we see improvement in the psychological consequences associated with ED, and the physical results of oxygenation and improved circulation as well as improved elasticity of penile tissue. ICP is effective 98 percent of the time.

It is important to mention again that ED is a progressive problem that will get worse if not treated effectively. Failure to treat will cause irreversible damage with worsening outcomes.

I encourage every man to seek treatment until success is realized. You deserve proper treatment. Please know that you are not alone. PE and ED are epidemic. More than fifty percent of men experience these problems, many suffering in silence or worse, not treated or handled appropriately when they do seek care.

Understand that rehabilitation is possible when treatment modalities are combined. It is important that protocols are designed by a skilled physician and proper patient follow-up and ongoing monitoring is applied.

WARNING: Surgical Penile Implants should be avoided unless all other treatments have been explored. Please understand, I am grateful for this option, but I feel that it is too often presented to the patient as the *only* option. I have successfully treated men with ICP and PRP that came to me for consultation after they were advised that the penile implant was the best choice. Penile implantation is not typically reversible and as with any surgery, has risks. If the surgical implant is your best option, make sure you have the penile implant surgery performed by a skilled urologist who performs these procedures on a very regular basis. This is important since these special surgeons have a much lower complication rate than the average urologist.

Tools: Treatment & Assistance

There are several tools and devices that prove useful in the pursuit of a fully satisfying sexual experience for both men and women. Some of these tools can be used during sexual intercourse, while others can be used to augments sexual arousal and vaginal or penile function and rehabilitation.

Penile Pumps/Vacuum Devices

A penile pump is a treatment option to enhance erectile function that works by forcing blood flow through the penis by negative pressure. The pump is constructed of a plastic tube that fits over the penis, a hand, battery or electric powered pump attached to the tube, and sometimes augmented by a band that fits around the base of the penis when erect.

Penile pumps have proven highly effective at helping men produce erections for sex, and since they do not require surgery, they are generally considered a non-invasive treatment procedure. This pump has helped men regain erectile functions after prostate surgery or radiation treatments. It has also been known to help patients with certain diseases maintain the length and girth of their penises.

Pumps are typically considered safe, but some risks or side effects do exist. Men can be at risk of bleeding if they are taking a blood thinning medication while using a pump. It is not safe to use if he has been diagnosed with sickle cell anemia or another blood disorder. Other issues can involve numbness, bruising, soreness, or feeling of "trapped" semen. Some men complain that their erections feel unnatural or that the penal pump can be awkward to use.

Your doctor might recommend a prescribed model of penis pump, but there are ones that are available without a prescription. Still, you should consult a doctor before deciding which one to purchase. Mayo Clinic recommends that you select one with a vacuum limiter, which keeps pressure from getting too high and injuring your penis.

The first step in using a penis pump is to place the plastic tube over your penis. Then you use a hand or electric pump attached to the tube to create a vacuum inside the tube and pull blood into the penis, creating an erection. Once you have an erection, you slip a rubber constriction ring around the base of your penis to help maintain the erection by keeping blood inside the penis.

Finally, you remove the vacuum device and proceed with sexual intercourse. Experts say that once you are used to using the pump, it will take about three minutes to obtain an erection. They advise that you do not leave the tension ring in place for more than 30 minutes, as cutting off the blood flow to your penis could cause damage.

According to MedicineNet.com, studies show that 50 to 80 percent of men are satisfied with the results of penal pumps (or vacuum devices). The device can prove useful for men who cannot seek hormone treatment or oral medications. They are particularly good for patients with poor blood flow to the penis, diabetes, depression or anxiety, and men who have had surgery for prostate or colon cancer.

Of course, the downside of using a penile pump — or the previously mentioned injection — is that it is cumbersome to do prior to a romantic encounter. This is one of the reasons why men seek the help of oral medications as that is a far more private approach to preparing for sex. However, if medications do not work and the idea of using a pump or injection for every sexual experience does not appeal to you, PRP treatments can help.

Vibrators

Stimulation of a woman's clitoris is a significant part of her arousal stage during sex. In fact, many women report only being able to orgasm through clitoral stimulation. Therefore, if a couple is open to the use of sexual devices, adding a vibrator to the foreplay portion of their sexual relations can help a woman achieve arousal and orgasm.

Kegel Devices

Kegel exercises are recommended for pregnant women to improve their ability to rebound from vaginal births. Other women practice Kegel exercises just to enhance their sexual function. But for women who unable to flex their muscles themselves, they are Kegel devices that can help with this exercise regimen.

Kegel exercisers are considered a solid solution for preventing or overcoming pelvic floor disorders and helping women gain pelvic strength in an easy and comfortable way. Kegel spherical shaped weights can be positions naturally to help a woman flex her muscles around the object. The weighted inner ball also offers resistance needed to strengthen and confirm placement.

Kegel exerciser products come in multiple resistance levels for women at different stages of pelvic strength and exercise routines. The exercises involve contracting the pelvic floor muscles, holding the contraction for several sections while taking deep breaths, releasing the contraction -then resting slightly before repeating the process. The Laselle™ routine for Kegel exercises recommends performing a Kegel set (10 repetitions) three times a week to strengthen pelvic floor muscles until the woman is ready for a higher level of resistance (**www.intimina.com**).

I have utilized several devices in my practice. To learn more, visit my website: **www.DoctorsStudio.com**.

In Office Electro-Stimulation for Pelvic Bowl Muscle Rehabilitation

In some instances, treatment for sexual dysfunction can involve electrical stimulation where electrodes are temporarily inserted into the rectum or vagina. The electrodes are then used to stimulate and strengthen pelvic floor muscles. This can be an effective treatment strategy, but it may take several months to fully realize the benefits.

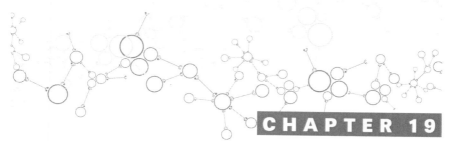

CHAPTER 19

Using PRP with Other Treatments

I feel confident in saying that PRP therapy is not always an effective stand-alone treatment for individuals looking to resolve their sexual problems. However, blending PRP therapies with other treatment strategies will improve the overall effectiveness of all medicines involved.

For example, PRP therapy will have benefits for men and women experiencing andropause or menopause, but not as much as if they are not hormonally balanced. The tremendous success reported in this book are based on individuals being hormonally correct.

There are other aspects that improve PRP therapy. Two of the most important are tools my patients use once they have received the O-Shot™ or Priapus Shot™.

The Priapus Shot™ and Other Treatments

In order for a man to receive the optimal benefit from PRP therapy, he needs to use a penile pump for several weeks after the treatment is administered. This will ensure that the PRP spreads throughout the penile region and stimulates the rejuvenation of the cells. The use of a penile pump will not only improve the results from PRP therapy, it will also elongate the benefits of the Priapus Shot™.

In addition to the penile pump, I may also recommend pairing the Priapus Shot™ with a different injectable treatment that will help men achieve an erection for a certain period of time. This ensures that the penis is properly stimulated and functioning while the PRP healing takes place. Penis function is one of those "use it or loss it" body parts, so it is important to achieve and maintain erections as quickly and as often as possible while the rejuvenating effects of PRP go to work.

I have even had patients who were in such a degenerative state that the PRP therapy was used so they could see benefits of oral medications. While on-going PRP therapy might enable them to achieve sexual function without medication, at least they are able to engage in sexual activity without the stress of having nothing work for them.

The O-Shot™ and Other Treatments

Outside of bio-identical hormone treatments, the most important combination for women might be using Kegel devices with the O-Shot™. While there are plenty of instructions for women on how to do Kegel exercises, I find that few women really know how to do the exercise properly. Furthermore, most women do not know they are doing the exercise wrong until they use a Kegel device and feel what the contraction is supposed to feel like.

I cannot emphasize enough the importance of women strengthening their pelvic floor. This will help a woman to continue to achieve orgasms as well as fend off incontinence. Women should begin and maintain Kegel exercises from the time they decide to have children through menopause and beyond. For this reason, all my patients have a Kegel device, whether they come to me for the O-Shot™ or just bio-identical hormone treatments.

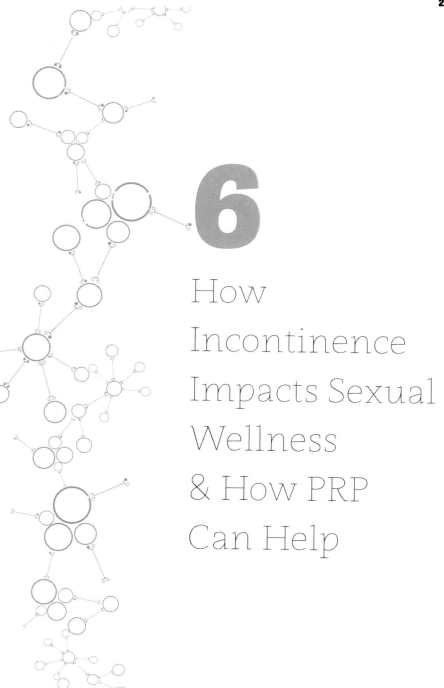

6

How
Incontinence
Impacts Sexual
Wellness
& How PRP
Can Help

Incontinence impacts all areas of a woman's life, sexually in particular. PRP has proven to be tremendously beneficial in treating female stress incontinence.

As shown in a previous diagram, the urethra is in close proximity to the vagina. What impacts a woman sexually often impacts the ability to control her bladder and vice versa. Healing one concern will likely have a positive effect on the other.

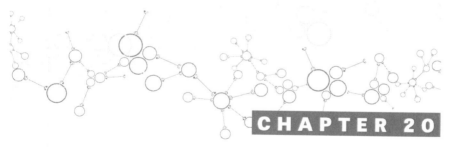

CHAPTER 20

Urinary Incontinence Defined

Urinary incontinence is defined as any involuntary leakage of urine, from small amounts when an individual laughs or coughs to a complete inability to control the bladder. The condition is typically broken down into two categories: Stress incontinence and Urge incontinence. Stress incontinence is caused when a person leaks urine in small doses due to laughter or other body reactions. Urge incontinence (or overactive bladder) is caused by muscle spasms. Other incontinence conditions include mixed, structural, and transient.

This might seem like an unrelated topic to that of sexual dysfunction, but in reality, the physiological closeness of a woman's urinary system to her sexual organs means that one can easily impact the other. Sadly, the embarrassment and decrease in self-confidence caused by urinary incontinence can negatively impact a woman's view of herself. Furthermore, incontinence in women can often lead to a decrease in independence, depression, and other negative feelings that make it difficult for women to feel "sexy."

Urinary incontinence is not a condition in and of itself, but a result of an underlying – often treatable – medical condition. Yet the symptom remains under-reported to medical practitioners. This might be because women think they have no other option but to wear "adult diapers," however, there are often other solutions depending on the cause. Most incontinence can be classified in one of two categories: Stress Incontinence and Urge Incontinence.

Stress incontinence is often caused by loss of support of the urethra. This condition typically occurs as a consequence of damage to pelvic support structures, which is a common result of childbirth.

Urge incontinence is caused by uninhibited contractions of the detrusor muscle. When these contractions occur, the individual leaks large amounts of urine or experiences insufficient warning to get to the bathroom in time.

Forty-three percent of women ages 30-80 report urinary incontinence to interfere with their daily activities

Coital Incontinence

Now that we have defined to two major types of incontinence, there is a third condition known as coital incontinence that I want to focus on for the purpose of this book. Coital incontinence is urinary leakage that occurs during penetration or orgasm (with a sexual partner or during masturbation). It has been reported in ten to twenty-four percent of sexually active women with pelvic floor disorders, according to a study by Matthew Karlovsky in 2010 (Karlovsky 2010).

In this paper, Karlovsky reports that only three percent of women self-report sexual disorders including coital incontinence and even with direct questioning, only twenty percent will admit to the condition. This condition more commonly occurs with penetration than with orgasm. Uro-dynamic testing shows that penetration is strongly correlated with stress urinary incontinence while orgasm more strongly correlated with detrusor over-activity.

Depending on the type of coital incontinence a woman reports, several methods have been suggested, from pharmacological to pelvic floor muscle retraining. Seeking treatment for this form of incontinence is particularly important for women because it is not as easy to hide as mild stress incontinence and cannot be dealt with by wearing a panty liner. While most forms of incontinence can be considered a personal issue, coital incontinence will have negative impact on a woman's sexual well-being and overall relationship with her partner.

Who is Effected by Incontinence

Bladder symptoms can affect women of all ages, but are more prevalent as a woman ages. Up to 35 percent of women over the age of 60 are estimated to have bladder control issues, according a Norwegian study in 2000 (Hannestad).

The authors found women suffer from the condition twice as often as men.

So while all women are at risk to experience incontinence, there are preventative measures. Bladder control dysfunction in women are frequently tied to obesity and diabetes and tend to increase as activity levels decrease. According to a 1997 study on nursing home admissions, 50 percent of nursing facility admissions are related to incontinence (Thom, DH).

Men tend to experience incontinence less often than women, due to the structure of the male urinary track. Typically, men who experience incontinence find it's related to conditions such as prostate cancer and the coinciding treatment. Other conditions such as strokes, multiple sclerosis, and congenital defects can affect male bladder control.

Physical & Psychological Effects of Incontinence

It is easy to see how incontinence can contribute to decreased self-confidence, depression, and decreased quality of life. It can also cause a person to avoid activities where they seem to experience the most severe loss of bladder control or social settings altogether. Studies have shown that there is a clear link between incontinence in women and depression. An article published in *Obstetrics & Gynecology* in 2005 surveyed nearly 6,000 women between the ages of 30 and 90. They found that in women experiencing incontinence the likelihood to be diagnosed with depression increased threefold (Melville).

The physical impact of incontinence begins with the need to plan ahead for any potential accidents or sadly, to clean one up. But the fear of an embarrassing incident can limit sexual experiences, physical activity, and social living for women. Ironically, maintaining a healthy weight and exercise has been shown to have a positive impact over bladder control, so the fear of physical activity caused by incontinence can lead to a negative health spiral if women do not seek treatment.

Why Seek Treatment/Types of Treatment

Women (and to some degree men) likely believe the only solution for incontinence is "adult diapers" but a consultation with a medical professional can open up other solutions. Treatment options range from bladder retraining to medications to pelvic floor therapy or surgery. There is also an innovative new treatment for incontinence that is based on platelet-rich plasma therapy.

A full exploration of this new treatment and how it is working as both a preventative measure and a treatment to existing bladder control issues will be explained. There are options beyond "living with" the condition. Finding a solid solution can help a woman regain her desire for an active social life and sexual intimacy. These are important parts of the quality of life for any age, but they are especially important for an older woman needing to maintain a healthy outlook on life. Addressing this issue is doubly important for anyone battling a life-threatening disease as the right mental outlook could prove vital to treatment success.

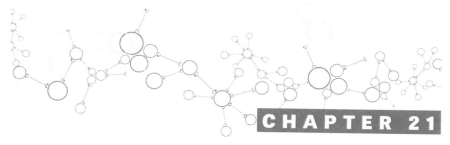

CHAPTER 21
Causes of Incontinence

Since urinary incontinence is not a disease, but rather a symptom, there are several underlying medical conditions or physical challenges that could be at the root of this problem. A comprehensive evaluation by a doctor is the best way to determine the source of incontinence, but this chapter will present a few possible explanations.

Causes of Temporary Incontinence

It is important to recognize that not all incontinence is a lingering condition. Temporary incontinence can be experienced as a result of certain foods, drinks, or medications that can impede natural bladder release functions.

Alcohol and Caffeine

Alcohol and caffeine both act as bladder stimulants and diuretics which can cause a persistent, frequent need to urinate or a sudden urge to go.

Bladder Irritation

In a related area, carbonated drinks, tea, and coffee (with or without caffeine) can cause bladder irritation and substances such as artificial sweetener, corn syrup, and certain foods/beverages that are high in spice content, sugar and acid, and citrus/tomatoes can negatively aggravate your bladder.

Urinary Tract Infection

Infections that irritate the bladder can cause a strong urge to urinate. Possible symptoms of a UTI also include burning sensations upon urination and foul-smelling urine.

Constipation

The rectum is located near the bladder and shares many of the same nerves as the bladder. Therefore, when a patient has a hard, compacted stool in their rectum, it can cause nerves to be overactive and increase urinary frequency. This situation can interfere with emptying of the bladder and cause overflow incontinence.

Persistent Urinary Incontinence

No matter the form of urinary incontinence (urge, stress, or other) the frequency should help determine if it is temporary or persistent. Factors that could cause a woman to have an on-going problem with urinary incontinence include:

Pregnancy & Childbirth

Pregnant women may experience stress incontinence as hormones change weight is gained for the enlarging uterus. Additionally, the stress of a vaginal delivery can weaken muscles needed for bladder control. Changes that occur during natural childbirth can also result in damage to the bladder nerves and supportive tissue.

Changes with Aging

Aging of the bladder muscle leads to a decrease in the bladder's capacity to store urine and increase overactive bladder symptoms; risk of overactive bladder increases in the presence of any blood vessel disease.

Menopause/Hysterectomy

After menopause women produce less estrogen. Estrogen keeps the lining of the bladder and urethra healthy. With less estrogen being produced, tissue around the urethra might become damaged and deteriorated and lead to incontinence.

For women who have experienced a hysterectomy, the muscles and ligaments that support the bladder can be damaged during the process of removing the uterus. In fact, any surgery that involves the reproductive system can damage the pelvic floor and lead to incontinence.

Painful Bladder Syndrome

This is a chronic condition that causes painful and frequent urination and possibly urinary incontinence.

Bladder Cancer/Stones or Prostate Cancer

In men, stress and urge incontinence can be associated with untreated prostate cancer as well as treatment (surgery or radiation) for the condition. Incontinence, urinary urgency, and burning with urination can be signs and symptoms of bladder cancer and stones. Other signs include blood in the urine and pelvic pain.

Neurological Disorders

Several diseases that impact brain waves and coordination can negatively impact quality of life and create incontinence. These conditions include Multiple Sclerosis, Parkinson's Disease, stroke, brain tumor, and spinal cord injury.

Obstruction

A tumor in the urinary track can block the normal flow of urine and as a result, cause incontinence. Urinary stones can form in the bladder and are often blamed for urinary leakage. These stones can present themselves in the kidney, bladder, or urethras.

Risk or Contributing Factors

Certain stages or conditions attribute to incontinence. Several risk or contributing factors include sex, age, weight, smoking, and other diseases. Please consider the following carefully.

Pregnancy

Any damage during natural childbirth can cause a woman to be more likely to experience stress incontinence as she ages. This probability increases depending on the number of pregnancies.

Age

As a woman ages, the bladder and urethra muscles lose some of their strength. Physical changes with age reduce the amount of liquid a bladder can hold while increasing the chances of involuntary urine release.

Weight

Being obese or overweight increase the pressure on a woman's bladder and surrounding muscles. The muscles are weakened and urine leaks out during a cough or sneeze.

Smoking

A chronic cough associated with smoking can lead to episodes of incontinence or aggravated incontinence. This cough puts stress on a woman's urinary sphincter and can lead to many cases of stress incontinence. Smoking might also increase the risk of overactive bladder by causing bladder contractions.

As stated before, incontinence seems to be a symptom rather than a disease. Talking to your doctor about the condition is very important. It will allow you to pinpoint the cause and seek proper treatment.

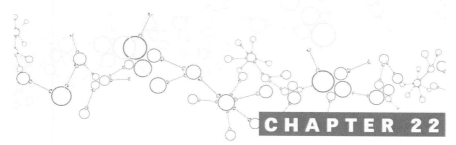

CHAPTER 22

PRP & Other Options for Incontinence Treatment

Treatment for urinary incontinence depends on the type of incontinence the women is experiencing, the severity of her issue, and the underlying medical cause for the incontinence. Generally speaking, doctors try the least invasive treatment techniques at first and then move onto other treatments, if necessary. As you look to address this problem with your doctor, he or she might recommend any of the following strategies alone or in cooperation with each other:

Behavioral Techniques

Bladder training is recommended as a means to control urge incontinence. It involves learning to delay urination until after the urge hits with the goal being to lengthen the time between trips to the bathroom.

Another strategy might involve putting your bladder on a schedule instead of waiting for the urge to go. The goal again is to extend bathroom trips to every couple of hours with the confidence that you have emptied your bladder in between trips.

Finally, like children who should not drink liquid before bed-time, you can work on limiting and managing your liquid intakes. In particular, you might want to cut back on alcohol, caffeine, and acidic foods, particularly late at night. Reducing your fluid intake while working to lose weight can eliminate bladder issues altogether (**www.mayoclinic.com**).

Exercises

Pelvic floor muscle exercises are used to strengthen the urinary sphincter and the muscles that control urination (Kegel exercises). This regimen is performed by squeezing the muscles used to stop from urinating and then holding the muscle contraction for several seconds. While it can be difficult to know if you are doing Kegel exercises properly, you can work with your doctor or use exercise weights that help you master the skill.

Electrical stimulation as described in the previous chapter to treat sexual dysfunction can also be used to correct stress, urge, and coital incontinence. When electrodes are inserted into a patient's rectum or vagina, they electrically stimulate and strengthen a woman's pelvic floor muscles. The procedure is done gently over a period of several months, but can produce solid, long-lasting results.

Medications

There are several prescription medications in the anticholinergics family that can calm an overactive bladder. Examples include the following:

- Oxybutynin (Ditropan)
- Tolterodine (Detrol)
- Darifenacin (Enablex)
- Fesoterodine (Toviaz)
- Solifenacin (Vesicare)
- Trospium (Sanctura)

Possible side effects of these medications are relatively minor; dry mouth, constipation, blurred vision, and flushing.

Other medical treatments include low-dose, topical estrogen and some antidepressants (though these present other possible side-effects).

Medical Devices

In some more serious cases, medical devices can be used to treat incontinence. These include urethral inserts which resemble a tampon and are equally disposable. These inserts are used for a specific activity or throughout the day to act as a plug and prevent leakage. They are not meant to be worn for long periods of time and are available only by prescription. This could be a helpful approach for dealing with coital incontinence during sex, but I believe some more natural solutions are best.

Your doctor might also prescribe you a Pessary, which is a stiff ring inserted in the vagina and worn all day. Since the bladder is located near the vagina, this device helps hold bladder and prevents leakage. The device must be removed and cleaned regularly and works well for patients with a dropped bladder or uterus.

Surgery

If any of the above treatments do not work or fail to work adequately, a doctor might recommend surgery. I sincerely want to help my patients avoid this radical treatment because of the potential issues that can arise during a surgical procedure. Some women developed their sexual dysfunction or incontinence problems because of surgeries. However, commonly used surgical procedures include following:

Sling Procedure: uses strips of your body's tissue and synthetic material to create a pelvic swing around the bladder neck and urethra. The sling helps keep the urethra closed when a woman coughs or sneezes.

Bladder Neck Suspension: is designed to provide support for your urethra and bladder neck, an area of thickened muscle where the bladder meets the urethra. It requires an abdominal incision so it is done with either general or spinal anesthesia.

Artificial Urinary Sphincter: is a small device for men who have weakened urinary sphincters from prostate cancer treatment or enlarged prostate glands. It is implanted around the man's bladder to keep the sphincter shut until he is ready to urinate. To empty his bladder, a man needs to press a valve implanted under his skin that cases the ring to deflate and allows urine to flow.

Any — or all — of these treatments can help you deal with urinary incontinence, but I believe curing it is a more beneficial strategy for total wellness. PRP treatments used to mend and strengthen urinary tissue and muscle can achieve just that. Please read on to see how PRP treatment works well with other more conventional approaches to address incontinence and sexual dysfunction.

PRP Therapy for Treatment of Incontinence

As mentioned before, the O-Shot™, which is a PRP treatment used for sexual dysfunction in women, has also proven successful in relieving issues related to incontinence. Some women have even been able to go off their medication for incontinence after receiving the O-Shot™. This treatment has proven beneficial for both stress and urge incontinence and most importantly, coital incontinence.

As with other PRP treatments, when the O-Shot™ is being used to treat incontinence, blood is drawn from the patient and placed in a processing unit that separates platelets, white blood cells, and serum from red blood cells. The white blood cells and platelets are concentrated and collected into a sterile syringe and then activated for treatment.

The O-Shot's™ rejuvenating capabilities help correct incontinence without the need for invasive surgery because it can help strengthen the muscles that cause stress incontinence. When injected, the PRP activates stem cells in the localized region while allowing the muscle tissues to rejuvenate and improve strength and ability to decrease urine flow.

A Few "Thinking Outside of the Box" Treatment Options to Improve Female Sexual Response

The very first treatment for women who suffer with low sex drive, difficulty with arousal and orgasm or lack of sexual organ sensitivity must be testosterone. I have said it a few times in this book, and I will say it again. Testosterone is a very powerful and necessary part of female function.

Once testosterone is corrected toward the upper end of optimal levels, it is time to get creative. At a recent ISSWSH conference (International Society for the Study of Women's Sexual Health), there was serious discussion about the many ways that physicians can help women restore pleasurable sexual response. Here are a few you may want to ask your doctor about. But don't be surprised if your doctor isn't aware of these treatments. You will want to find a physician who focuses of helping women with sexual issues.

1. Testosterone — First Line Therapy

    a. Dopamine Agonists like Cabergoline 0.5mg twice a week. This will lower prolactin and help women with ease of orgasm.

2. Wellbutrin 75mg-150mg daily. I know that it is a commonly used antidepressant but its mechanism of action is to stimulate dopamine, which stimulates sexual desire.

3. Oxytocin either injectable 10iu, lozenge 250iu, or nasal spray 60-120iu to significantly improve sexual response in women who are having difficult reaching climax.

4. Progesterone 200-1000mg in capsule form a few hours prior to sex has pro-sexual benefits.

BONUS GIFT: Studio Solution 4-Phase Program

To download the pdf, visit my website: DoctorsStudio.com.
Under Nutrition, enter the code "Book."

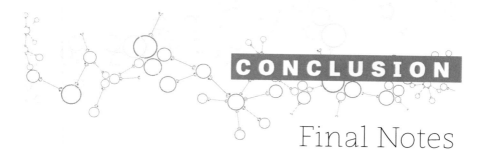

CONCLUSION

Final Notes

This book is written and medications are being pushed through the FDA because of the serious need for effective treatments. I am very proud of Dr. Runels and many other physicians who have faced criticism and have continued on, working collaboratively with the focus on helping patients. As a group, we share and inspire each other as we discover new ways to apply PRP technology.

If you are challenged by sexual changes and/or urinary incontinence, I hope this book has inspired you to seek help. If you are a physician, I hope you are inspired to be a partner in helping men and women find their way back to optimal function. I can tell you that the journey is rewarding and impactful.

Sexual desire, sexual function, sexual satisfaction and intimacy are central to human vitality, confidence and sense of self for men and women, both young and old. It is not the only thing that is important to health and vitality of course, but it is very important. I hope this conversation continues and that medical pioneers are embraced and encouraged to continue their work.

I believe the innovative nature of PRP treatment in the form of O-Shot™ and Priapus Shot™ will tremendously improve the quality of life for many individuals of all ages. There is much about PRP that is **not** covered in this book. We are finding new and beneficial uses for PRP every day. I personally have helped women with lichen sclerosis, interstitial cystitis, vulvodynia, pain with intercourse, acne, facial rejuvenation, restoration of breasts and nipple sensitivity after breast augmentation and/or reconstruction, joint and muscle pain and men with Peyronie's disease, painful ejaculation, and pain after trauma to the scrotum.

As much as I want to make the public aware of these treatment options, I also want to promote the training to other doctors.

You can visit Join.StudioPRP.com to find a physician training workshop that works best for you. We now have physicians of all specialties offering training and sharing valuable insight.

I encourage you to "think outside the box", never give up, never stop caring about each other and share what you have with the world. We all have enormous gifts to offer.

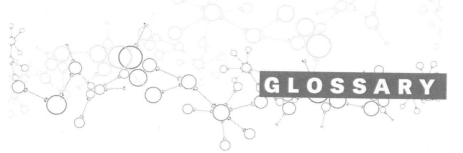

GLOSSARY

Andropause: A set of effects that appears in some aging men which superficial similarities to menopause in women.

Bio-Identical Hormone Therapy (BHRT): A term that refers to the use of hormones that are identical, on a molecular level, with hormones your body produces naturally.

Clitoris: A part of a woman's sexual organ that is a complex of sensitive tissue consisting of both visible and nonvisible components. The visible component is known as the glans; a sensitive bulb of soft tissue located at the junction of the labia minora (small lips). The non-visible components extend deep into the body and is associated to the lateral walls for the vagina and deep to the vulva.

Growth Factors: Various proteins that promote the growth, organization, and maintenance of cells or tissue. Some of these factors are responsible for attracting stem cells, regenerating nerves, growing new blood vessels, healing wounds, stimulating collagen, etc.

Incontinence: An inability to restrain natural discharges of urine. Stress Incontinence (SUI) caused by pressure of coughing, sneezing, jumping, laughing, etc. Urge Incontinence is the sudden urge to urinate with the inability to restrain. A person can have one or both types of incontinence.

Kegel exercises: An exercise performed to strengthen muscles of the pelvic floor. Strengthening these muscles is important to overall vaginal health, urinary continence and sexual function and satisfaction.

Libido: Sexual instinct or sex drive. Desire to engage is sexual play.

Menopause: The period of time after a woman stops menstruating for more than 12 months.

Periurethral: The space between the urethra and the vaginal wall. This space contains the Skene's glands, many blood vessels, and sensory nerves.

Skene's Glands: Glands that are located on the anterior wall of the vagina near the end of the urethra. These glands are surrounded with tissue that reaches up inside the vagina and swells with blood during sexual arousal.

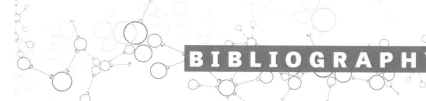

BIBLIOGRAPHY

Alexander, Brian, "Sorry Guys: Up to 80% of Women Admit Faking It," www.nbcnews.com. June 30, 2010.

Carroll, Will, "Is PRP Therapy, Used by Alex Rodriguez and Zack Greinke, Miracle or Mirage?" www.blecherreport.com. July 8, 2013.

Case-Lo, Christine, "Hair Loss and Testosterone," www.healthline.com. September 23, 2013.

Clarke, Suzan, "Pink Viagra? Drug Promises to Boost Female Sex Drive," www.abcnews.go.com. May 25, 2010.

Esposito K., Ciotola M. et al. "Hyperlipidemia and sexual function in pre-menopausal women," Journal of Sexual Medicine (6): 1696-1703 (2009).

Gleason, Joseph, Slezak, Jeffrey, Jung, Howard, et al. "Regular Nonsteroidal Anti-Inflammatory Drug Use and Erectile Dysfunction," The Journal of Urology (Vol 185): 1388-1393 (2011).

Gravina GL, Brandetti F, Martini P, et al. "Measurement of the Thickness of the Urethrovaginal Space in Women with or without Vaginal Orgasm," *Journal of Sexual Medicine* (3): 610-618. 2008.

Hannestad, Yngvild, Rortveit, Guri, Sandvic, Hogne, Hunskaar, Steinar, "A community-based epidemiological survey of female urinary incontinence." Journal of Clinical Epidemiology (Vol. 53): 1150-1157 (2000).

Harris, Lindsay N. and Larson, Andrew I. "Platelet-Rich Plasma Accelerates Healing," Aspen Orthopaedic Associates and Aspen Sports Medicine Foundation (2009).

Horst, Van Der, Stuebinger, Henrik, Seif, Christoph, et. al, "Priapism – Etiology, Pathophysiology and Management," *International Brazilian Journal of Urology* (Vol 29): 391-400 (2003).

Hurlemann R, Patin A, Onur OA, Cohen MX, Baumgartner T, Metzler S, Dziobek I, Gallinat J, Wagner M, Maier W, Kendrick KM (April 2010). "Oxytocin enhances amygdala-dependent, socially reinforced learning and emotional empathy in humans". *J. Neurosci.* **30** (14): 4999–5007.

Irani, J., Salomon L., Oba R., Bouchard P., Mottet N., "Efficacy of venafaxine, medroxyprogesterone acetate, and cyproterone acetate for the treatment of vasomotor hot flashes in men taking gonadotropin-releasing hormone analogues for prostate cancer: a double-blind, randomized trial," Lancet Oncology (2): 147-154 (2009).

James, Susan Donaldson, "Female Orgasm May be Tied to 'Rule of Thumb'" www.abcnews.go.com. September 4, 2009.

Karlovsky, Matthew E. "Female Urinary Incontinence During Sexual Intercourse (Coital Incontinence): A Review," *The Female Patient* (34): 32-36 (2009).

Kilchevsky A, Vardi Y, Lowenstein L, Gruenwald I., "Is the Female G-Spot Truly a Distinct Anatomic Entity?" *The Journal of Sexual Medicine,* 2012.

Laumann Eo, Paik A, Rosen RC. "Sexual dysfunction in the United States: prevalence and predictors." *Journal of the American Medical Association* (281): 537-544 (1999).

Melville, Jennifer L., Delany, Kristin, Newton, Katherine, and Katon, Wayne, "Incontinence Severity and Major Depression in Incontinent Women." Obstetrics & Gynecology (Vol 106: 3): 585-592, 2005.

Muehlenhard CL and Shippee SK, "Men's and women's reports of pretending orgasm." Journal of Sex Research (6): 552-567, 2010.

Niesen, Joan, "Platelet-Rich Plasma Therapy Big with Athletes," www.foxsportsnorth.com July 3, 2012.

Patel, Sandeep, Dhillon, Mandeep S., Aggarwal, Sameer, et al. "Treatment with Platelet-Rich Plasma is More Effective than Placebo for Knee Osteoarhritis," The American Journal of Sports Medicine (Vol 41): 356-364 (2013).

Podesta, Luga, Crow, Scott A., Volkmer, Dustin, et al. "Treatment of Partial Ulnar Collateral Ligament Tears in the Elbow with Platelet-Rich Plasma," American Journal of Sports Medicine (Vol 41): 1689-1694 (2013).

Ronbinson, Marnia, "Porn-Induced Sexual Dysfunction Is a Growing Problem," *Psychology Today* (2011).

Runels, Charles, *Activate the Female Orgasm System: The Story of the O-Shot*, 2013.

Schwarz, Alan, "A Promising Treatment for Athletes in Blood," *New York Times.* February 16, 2009.

Shomon, Mary, "Men: Is Your Thyroid Causing Sexual Problems?" thyroid.about.com. November 15, 2013.

Thom, DH, Haan, MN, Van Den Eeden, SK, "Medically recognized urinary incontinence and risks of hospitalizations, nursing home admission and mortality," *Age Ageing* (5): 367-374, 1997.

Waldinger, MD, Quinn, P, Dilleen, M, et al. "A Multinational Population Survey of Intravaginal Ejaculation Latency Time," *Journal of Sexual Medicine* (4): 492-497 (2005).

Wood, Samuel, "O-Shot May Improve Female Sexual Response," PR Newswire Services (2012).

2009 PRP applied to perineum post "crush injury" to simulate radical prostatectomy http://www.ncbi.nlm.nih.gov/pubmed/19151738

2012 The Neuroprotective Effect of Platelet-rich Plasma on Erectile Function in Bilateral Cavernous Nerve Injury Rat Model - http://www.jsm.jsexmed.org/article/S1743-6095%2815%2933795-4/pdf

2013 - Finally asking the question about "optimized PRP" and realizing better results: http://www.ncbi.nlm.nih.gov/pubmed/23950105

Asian Journal of Andrology (2009): 215–221 A Pilot Study of the Effect of Localized Injections of Autologous Platelet Rich

Plasma (PRP) for the Treatment of Female Sexual Dysfunction Charles Runels*, Hugh Melnick, Ernest Debourbon and Lisbeth Roy Medical School, Birmingham, Alabama, USA

Runels et al., J Women's Health Care 2014, 3:4 http://dx.doi.org/10.4172/2167-0420.1000169

Skenes Glands: https://www.netterimages.com/order-confirmation.htm

Female Urinary System: http://www.istockphoto.com/vector/female-urinary-system-gm475982765-26188045?st=e3f799e

Maslow Hierarchy of Needs photo: http://www.123rf.com/profile_pytyczech

Exchange the Anatomy of the Penis from Shutterstock to http://www.netterimages.com

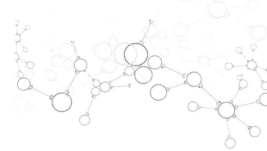

Q

Quality of life, 281, 161, 163, 165, 180, 190, 206, 224, 236, 60, 264, 265, 270, 82, 92, 115, 116, 22, 24, 25, 28, 32, 102, 119, 214, 7

R

Regenerate, 35, 44, 216, 58, 136, 139, 21, 29

Regenerative, 35, 39, 40, 46, 166, 168, 244, 51, 53, 57, 62, 72, 74, 81, 84, 86, 87, 89, 95, 139, 18, 21-23, 27, 29, 31, 33, 214, 5

Rehabilitation, 166, 247-250, 254, 73, 82, 84, 86, 87, 108, 138, 22, 25, 30, 31

Rejuvenate, 35, 216, 50, 51, 278, 21, 26, 29

Relationships, 161, 162, 58, 60, 63, 108, 111-113, 26, 101, 102, 214

S

Sex, 285, 287, 279, 280, 38, 160, 161, 163, 164, 174-176, 179, 181, 183, 185-187, 190, 193, 197, 198, 206, 207, 209-211, 227, 229, 232, 236, 239, 243, 245, 246, 248, 251, 252, 54, 56, 60, 62, 63, 65, 67, 69, 271, 276, 73, 74, 76, 78, 83, 85, 88, 95, 103-110, 112, 113, 115, 121-124, 127-129, 131, 133, 139, 143, 150, 156, 157, 284, 28, 100-102, 119, 172, 7

Sexual Dysfunction, 287-289, 38, 44-46, 159-162, 164, 167, 168, 173, 174, 177, 181, 183, 185-188, 190, 193, 194, 198, 201, 203, 205, 209, 210, 222, 227, 238, 244, 254, 49, 53, 57, 59, 61, 62, 261, 274, 276, 277, 71, 72, 74, 75, 77-79, 81, 86, 91-95, 104, 108-114, 122, 124, 127-129, 137, 142, 146-149, 153, 17, 18, 21, 22, 25-31, 117-119, 171, 172, 214, 1, 2, 8, 9

Sexual dysfunction, 287-289, 38, 44-46, 159-162, 164, 167, 168, 173, 174, 177, 181, 183, 185-188, 190, 193, 194, 198, 201, 203, 205, 209, 210, 222, 227, 238, 244, 254, 49, 53, 57, 59, 61, 62, 261, 274, 276, 277, 71, 72, 74, 75, 77-79, 81, 86, 91-95, 104, 108-114, 122, 124, 127-129, 137, 142, 146-149, 153, 17, 18, 21, 22, 25-31, 117-119, 171, 172, 214, 1, 2, 8, 9